STRENGTH TRAINING FOR FASTER SWIMMING

DEDICATION
To William Anderson, who taught me by example what it means to be an athlete.

STRENGTH TRAINING FOR FASTER SWIMMING

by Blythe Lucero

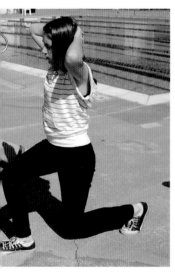
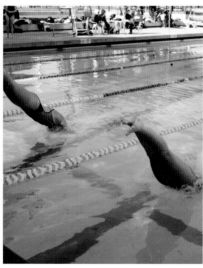
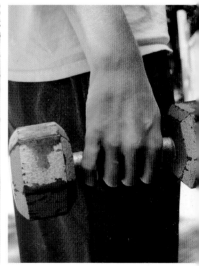

Meyer & Meyer Sport

British Library Cataloguing in Publication Data
A catalogue record for this book is available from the British Library

Strength Training for Faster Swimming
Maidenhead: Meyer & Meyer Sport (UK) Ltd., 2012
ISBN 978-1-84126-339-7

© 2012 by Meyer & Meyer Sport (UK) Ltd.
Auckland, Beirut, Budapest, Cairo, Cape Town, Dubai, Indianapolis,
Kindberg, Maidenhead, Sydney, Olten, Singapore, Tehran, Toronto
Member of the World
Sport Publishers' Association (WSPA)
www.w-s-p-a.org
Printed by: B.O.S.S Druck und Medien GmbH
ISBN 978-1-84126-339-7
E-Mail: info@m-m-sports.com
www.m-m-sports.com

TABLE OF CONTENTS

INTRODUCTION

As swimmers, we appreciate what an amazing thing the human body is. After all, we use our bodies from head to toe to perform our sport. The complex system of muscles that weaves together over our frames allows us to do the quick, explosive movements, and the long, repetitious movements that make up swimming. Our muscles work in tandem to make it possible to perform tasks as simple as putting on goggles and as lofty as winning Olympic gold.

Yet, when we see a fantastic swimmer moving through the water with grace and speed, we don't associate their speed with muscular strength. Instead we associate it with skill. We notice their skill at reducing drag and maintaining a streamlined body shape. We notice their skill at "feeling" the water and using it to their advantage. We notice their skill at coordinating stroke actions that together produce fluid forward motion.

In fact, it is widely accepted that swimming is not a matter of muscling your way through the water. Swimmers have to know how to swim!

Still, it is puzzling to see swimmers with such picture-perfect strokes that they could star in a video on stroke technique who, when the time comes to swim fast, are unable to generate speed. Then there are swimmers with equally developed stroke technique who move through the water with such velocity that they appear to be wearing invisible flippers. So, what is the difference? What makes one swimmer able to achieve speed in the water but another swimmer unable to?

The main difference is strength. The mechanics of swimming are not based on technique alone but also on the application of force and power. When we swim, our muscles are engaged in an integrated sequence of actions to both exert resistance on the water and to balance and stabilize our bodies so that forward motion is realized. In this way, when two swimmers, both with solid stroke technique, are swimming side by side, the stronger swimmer will be faster. Thus, that fantastic swimmer, who looks like poetry in motion, is in actuality muscling his way through the water! By adding strength to skill, faster swimming is possible.

As the title of this book suggests, strength training for swimming is a very specialized activity. The specific audience and the specific goal of this book lead us to the logical conclusion that swimming strength is not developed very well through a general approach to strength training. Building useable strength for swimming requires attention to more than making the muscles strong. It requires orientation toward specific aspects of strength. It requires simulation of swimming directionality and tempo. Above all, it requires attention to training multi-muscle movements, like those that make up swimming. General strength training may produce some positive results in a hit or miss fashion, but it can also produce bulk and fatigue that can interfere with swimming. To make sure that strength work produces the intended results for swimmers, it must be designed and structured with swimming in mind.

To illustrate this point, I would like to share a story that a swimmer recounted with me about the last year of his long swimming career. He told me that he had been a dedicated swimmer, with twelve years of training and competition experience under his belt. He had enviable technique, and even more enviable endurance. Knocking off 10 x 200 on the 2:30, and swimming double workouts five days a week, was no problem. He was, in fact, a coaches' ideal of self-motivation, and a role model of good work ethic to the rest of his team. He did it all because he dreamed of going to the Olympics. It was more than a dream though; it was a goal, and at the age of 18, he was determined to make the Olympic team.

After months of intense training, he found himself at a plateau and decided to supplement his swimming with weights. In addition to swimming over 80,000 each week, he also went to the gym and lifted weights, understanding that more strength would benefit his swimming speed. He developed a routine of exercises from those he observed other people at the gym doing regularly, including all the standard body building lifts. He did bench press, military press and French curls by the dozens. He got to the point that he could lift impressive amounts of weight with little effort. He continued this routine diligently for several months, building a large and well-defined upper body. As the last meet of the season approached, he found himself feeling quite tired, and his test swims were not outstanding, showing a sluggish tempo and higher stroke count than desirable. Still, going into the competition, he maintained his confidence. He believed that because he had worked as hard as he could both in and out of the water, he would make a swimming breakthrough. But after his race, he was stunned to have made no progress at all. In fact, he had clocked a time that he achieved two years before. Disappointed that all of his dedication and training had made no impact, he became disheartened and soon lost interest in swimming, allowing his dream to slip away.

This sad story is all too common. A swimmer with amazing work ethic and goal-oriented drive gets into a cycle of extreme over-training and non-specific, non-progressive strength training. Despite red flags – including plateau, fatigue, and reduced flexibility – that foretell poor race results, the swimmer keeps training and fails to reach the goal.

Coaches and swimmers: This is preventable!

This book addresses strength training as a means to achieve more speed in the water, rather than simply a means to become stronger. Emphasis is placed on both the underlying concepts and crucial details of building strength that transfers to swimming. Readers will explore how to structure a strength training program that will work with the swimming routine. Readers will learn about the importance of individualizing training to match a swimmer's stage of development, level of experience, and swimming specialty. Readers will discover what kinds of activities build usable strength in the water.

At the end of the book, a series of strength training routines and circuits are included for each stage of development. Before skipping right to that chapter, please take time to read the rest of the book first so you will have the background information that will prepare you to get the best results possible.

Here is to reaching your swimming dreams!

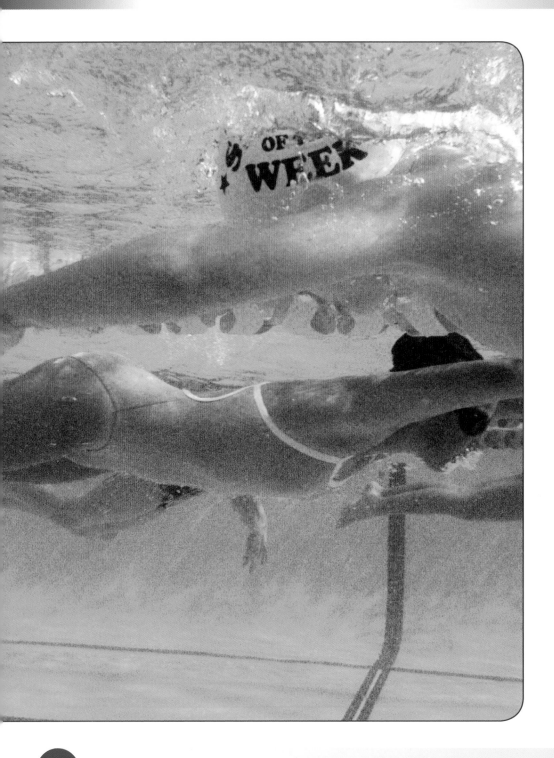

1 WHAT MAKES SWIMMERS FAST?

The common goal in competitive swimming is to swim faster and, to a large extent, training is the means to that objective. The evolution of our sport has been marked by countless theories of training, based on emerging science, past results and intuition. Determined swimmers pair with inspired coaches in search of the perfect formula for attaining swimming speed. Training methods using more volume, or less volume but more intensity both in and out of the water, diets with more protein or less protein, and various pre-competition rituals have been designed with the single purpose of defying speed barriers. And swimming times keep dropping, as many of these strategies have resulted in incredible success for individual swimmers. But the fact is no single training formula has worked across the board. Some swimmers do better swimming twice a day, while others only once. Some swimmers will benefit from weight training, while others will get more out of a self-resistance program. Some swimmers can eat anything, anytime, but some have to carefully watch their calorie intake. Some swimmers race better practicing all the way up to the day before the meet, but others need several days, or even weeks of rest.

We have come to understand that a uniform training strategy for competitive swimming is both ineffective and unrealistic. Differences in stage of development, conditioning and skill level, body type, rate of recovery, and swimming specialty reveal that an individualized approach to training yields the best results.

While there is no single alchemy, certain training principles have endured and gained acceptance as integral elements in the quest for swimming speed.

SWIMMING

The main element in a swimmer's training, at every stage of his or her career, must be swimming. Without frequent and ample time in the water, even the best athlete will not be prepared to swim fast because he will not be prepared to swim well. Only time in the water enables a swimmer to develop the swimming technique that leads to the essential ability to "feel" the water. Only time in the water teaches a swimmer to eliminate drag and be more "fishlike." Only time in the water gives a swimmer the experience of coordinating stroke actions and accessing the best sequence of muscles to accomplish fluid forward motion. Only time in the water enables a swimmer to practice stroke economy, balance and stability in the aquatic environment. There is no substitute for time in the water. To be a faster swimmer, one first has to be a good swimmer.

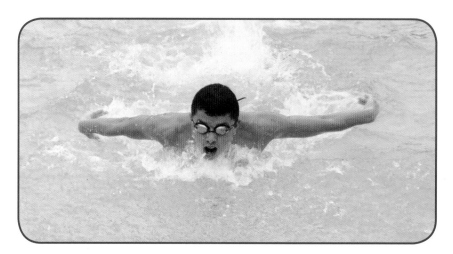

ATHLETIC BASE

The saying goes, "better athletes make better swimmers." There is no way around it. Swimming is not a sport that gives immediate gratification. When a person comes into competitive swimming without a base of athleticism, a great deal of time and energy must be devoted to building that base, to prepare the person to take on the rigors of training for competitive swimming. In contrast, when these qualities are already present, a swimmer is able to excel faster. A swimmer who comes into swimming with an athletic base in place is able to concentrate on developing solid swimming skills, gaining swimming experience, and swimming fast!

Athleticism is defined in many ways. For the purposes of this book, we will measure athleticism in the following terms:

1) **Cardiovascular fitness** — ability of the body to transport and utilize oxygen
2) **Flexibility** — range of motion
3) **Coordination** — integrating movements into unified effective effort
4) **Strength** — power, force, explosiveness and stability against resistance

An active lifestyle beginning in childhood that includes casual and organized activities that involve running, jumping, climbing and balancing builds overall athletic ability.

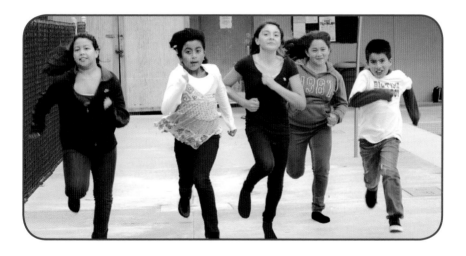

STRENGTH TRAINING

When analyzing the qualities of athleticism that are most developed by swimmers, we see that, without a doubt, competitive swimming provides some of the best cardiovascular fitness of any sport. The full body requirements and repetitive nature of our sport promotes high levels of aerobic capacity and cardiovascular efficiency, much like runners and cyclists possess, but with the added requirement of propelling ourselves through a medium thicker than air. Swimming also requires mastery of breathing timing (more so than any other sport). Whereas on land, athletes have no restrictions on breathing, in swimming getting new air is limited to the time when the face is out of the water, ultimately boosting fitness even further.

Swimmers are also very flexible, and in many cases, almost too flexible. The loose joints (especially in the shoulders) that enable a swimmer to reach and stroke effectively, and move so fluidly can also allow the bones to move around at the joint, causing inflammation and pain. The only area where swimmers often lack enough flexibility is at the ankle, where it is desirable to have the ability to easily point the toes and create a straight line to the knee. Still, among land athletes, only ballet dancers have better ankle flexibility than swimmers.

Swimmers are very coordinated, as well. The complex nature of swimming uses every part of the body to move forward in a series of movements within each stroke cycle, encouraging an intuitive understanding of the kinetic chain. And, in what other sport does the athlete propel himself or herself at full speed toward a wall, then tuck and reverse directions without slowing down?

Finally, we come to strength, the final measure of athletic condition. As we compare the strength developed by swimmers with the strength developed by other athletes, it is clear that swimmers do not develop the same degree of musculature as many other athletes. For example, football players and weightlifters develop more muscle bulk than swimmers in order to succeed in their sports. But since swimming does not have the same strength requirements as football and weightlifting, should we be concerned with strength levels in swimming? The answer is yes! While swimmers do not need muscle size to excel, they do need muscle strength.

There are four types of strength that swimmers should be concerned with:

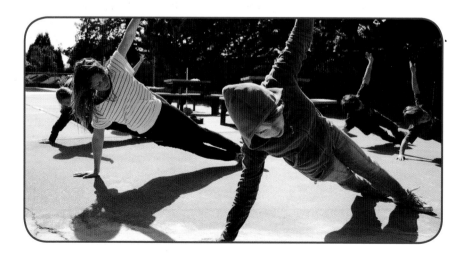

FORCE

Force is the maximum amount of resistance that can be applied. In the case of swimming, force refers to the maximum resistance that can be applied to the water, in one stroke, from the beginning of the catch through the end of the underwater stroke, accelerating from beginning to end. More deliverable force improves a swimmer's distance per stroke, ultimately producing more potential for speed.

POWER

Power is the ability to maintain force over time. In swimming, power is required to do the series of strokes it takes to complete any single lap or distance in the pool. A swimmer who is able to keep a higher percentage of force throughout his or her race all the way to the end with less fatigue is able to maintain more even splits, and therefore produce a faster overall time.

EXPLOSIVENESS

Explosiveness is the ability to recruit a burst of force. In swimming, explosiveness is beneficial for fast starts, turns and sprinting. A swimmer with good explosive strength is quick off the blocks and has turns that set him or her apart from the field. Explosiveness is also the basis of sprinting. However, it should be pointed out that swimming even the shortest race, with its 20 to 30-second average time span, takes more than just explosiveness, it also takes power and force to sprint well.

STABILITY

Stability refers to one's ability to balance and control movements from within the body. In swimming, we must be able to create and maintain integrity in motion, and do so without the support of the ground. The ability to stabilize oneself is crucial to producing forward motion while floating. A swimmer with good stability is able to generate power from the center of the body and send it upward to the arms and downward to the legs in a continual chain reaction to generate speed.

A carefully designed strength training program enhances a swimmer's water training, dramatically enriching its value. In addition to swimming, strength training that addresses all four kinds of strength should be considered an essential part of a swimmer's long-term training.

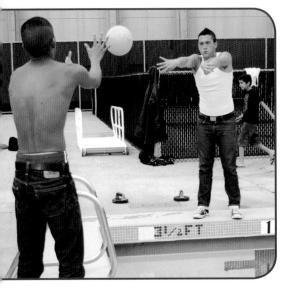

HOW LAND-BASED STRENGTH TRAINING ENCOURAGES SWIMMING SPEED

Resistance is the basis of all strength building. Although there are some effective ways of increasing resistance during swimming, including hand paddles, tethered swimming, drag suits and towing chutes and pails, the reality is that none of these methods can deliver the results in terms of building strength that can be achieved on land.

With more gravitational effect on land than in the water, more load is possible. Strategic strength training that develops the force required to resist a load on land builds the swimmer's ability to apply more force to the underwater stroke, both in the catch and the acceleration of the arm toward the finish, thus moving his or her body farther and faster per stroke with less fatigue. In addition to this, self-stabilization, especially in the horizontal swimming position, is much more challenging out of the water. By learning to maintain body position against gravity on land, a swimmer will develop a stronger foundation to swim from.

With less resistance in the air than in the water, the tempo of movements can be quicker on land. Strategic strength training that develops the power to repeatedly move a load through the air gives the swimmer more strength to overcome the thickness of the water. It also brings an increased and sustainable tempo to his or her swimming stroke. In addition, practicing true explosive actions on land gives a swimmer quicker reaction time to his or her starts, more speed off the walls in turns, and a solid base for sprinting.

By making use of gravity to increase load, and by making use of the "thin" environment of the air to increase rate, strength is developed better and faster on land than it would be in the water. Strength training on land increases force potential, improves core stability, builds deliverable power, and develops explosiveness, all of which positively encourage more speed and decrease fatigue in the water. A swimmer who uses the ideal environment to build strength brings an advantage back to the ideal environment for swimming.

WHY SWIMMING IS NOT ENOUGH

In the aquatic environment, resistance and gravity provide both challenges and advantages. These challenges make strength the most difficult athletic quality to develop through water training alone. The advantages make strength the least noticeable athletic quality in swimmers. Swimmers, in fact, are often are so developed in terms of fitness, flexibility and coordination that strength is overlooked.

Swimmers spend a great deal of time learning the essential skill of overcoming the resistance of the water. We search for the best body position so we will slide through the water without interrupting it, avoiding drag that will slow us down, much like an airplane that is designed to cut through the air with the least resistance. But in addition to learning to treat the water like air, we must also learn to treat it like rock. We must learn to use the resistance of the water to our advantage. We must be able to grab hold of it, like it was solid, anchoring our hand at a point in front of us, then move our body past that point, similar to a rock climber who grasps the rock at a point above, then lifts his or her body beyond that point.

Applying resistance to the water takes strength, and just like a more streamlined swimmer has an advantage, a stronger swimmer also has an advantage. But training in the water limits our ability to develop strength in two ways. First, the thickness of the water makes the rate of each motion to advance the body slower than it would on land. Second, in the reduced gravity environment of the water, the swimmer's body weight is lighter, which produces less load for the swimmer to move.

The obvious question that arises is: if our medium is water, why should we be concerned with moving at the rate we could on land, or being able to move a larger load than we need to in the water? The answer is, that when we are able to recruit more force, power, explosiveness and stability, in combination with using good swimming skills, we are able to achieve more speed in the water. Land-based strength training builds useable strength for swimmers. A training routine that combines swimming and strength work on land gives swimmers an edge over water-based training alone.

MORE BENEFITS OF STRENGTH TRAINING

While the primary objective for swimmers engaged in land-based strength training is to build more speed in the water, there are additional benefits as well.

INJURY PREVENTION

Strength training is one of the most proactive steps a swimmer can take to prevent injuries, especially to the shoulders. The recognizable physique of a swimmer features large shoulders and a well-developed upper body, but is often punctuated by poor posture. The shortened chest muscles and lengthened back muscles developed by swimmers can result in posture imbalance, often accompanied by shoulders that drop forward, and are sometimes internally rotated. Long-term swimming with this posture can lead to inflammation around the shoulders and pain when the bones are not held firmly in place on all sides. Eventually, if not corrected, such an imbalance can lead to injury that can take a swimmer out of action. Strength training can correct imbalances by targeting the stabilizing muscles around the shoulder joints. Posture can also be improved by targeting the muscles of the upper back. Balanced strength and better posture help a swimmer remain injury free.

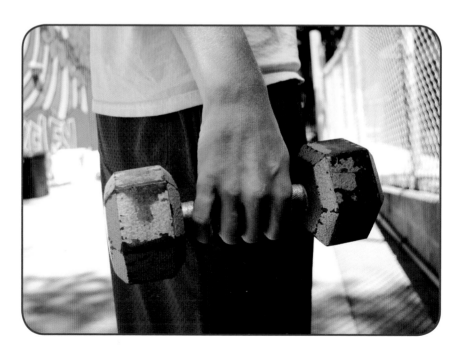

TRAINING TIME MANAGEMENT

Another benefit of strength training is the management of training time. Limitations on water time, as well as limits on the productive swimming a person can be expected to do in one session can lead to training content deficiencies. As we try to include every training element into our limited water time, we may end up short on every element. By supplementing water training with additional time dedicated to land-based strength work, more value can be achieved in with the overall training routine. Precious water time can be used to practice solid technique, including stroke coordination, the elimination of drag, refining "feel" for the water, and to experience swimming economically at any speed. Land work can be used to develop the full spectrum of swimming-specific strength, where it is developed most efficiently.

NEW FEEDBACK

Strength training also adds a new dimension of feedback to a swimmer's routine. It is common for swimmers to become so accustomed to swimming that they forget to pay attention to the mechanics of what they are doing in the water. Land-based strength training provides a new way to "connect" with the physical actions of the sport. In addition, swimmers can observe improvement in strength as they adapt to the workload. More repetitions, more resistance, and faster tempo achieved over time on land give a swimmer concrete feedback that they are improving, thereby building confidence and motivation.

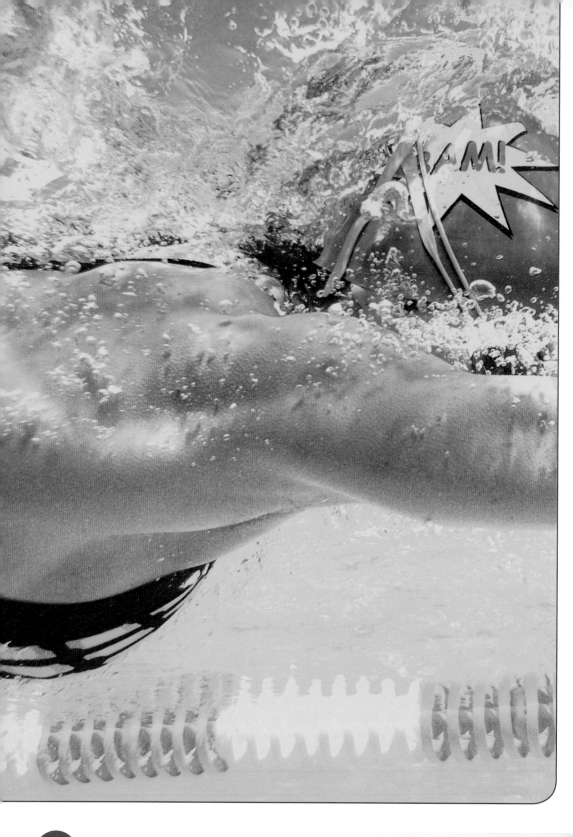

2 MAKING STRENGTH TRAINING COUNT

The ultimate effectiveness of a strength training program is measured in terms of what is accomplished in the pool. There must be positive results. To make sure this happens, the strength training program should be designed and redesigned to meet that objective. It should evolve as the swimmer's strength evolves and consider the individual swimmer's changing needs. This means that careful observation and monitoring must be an essential element of the program. By evaluating results, or lack of results, we can tailor the program to work better or take positive steps to redirect efforts. Ongoing evaluation should consider a number of issues, as outlined below.

TRANSFERABILITY

The key to a successful strength training program is that every activity must be transferable to swimming speed. If it doesn't transfer, then it is a waste of time, or worse, it could even hinder faster swimming. Every strength training exercise can make a swimmer tired, but once the swimmer recovers, does the new strength improve his or her swimming speed?

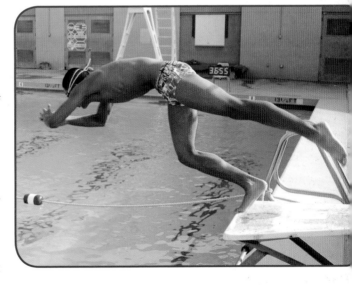

In order to get strength work to transfer to swimming speed, it is important to perform activities that use swimming-like movement and target major swimming-specific muscle groups that together produce that movement, including both visible and underlying muscles. We must strengthen the muscles that move us forward as well as those that stabilize us. It is important to consider directionality when applying resistance on land. Our primary effort should be focused in simulating the direction of swimming. It is also important to mimic swimming tempo as much as possible. A tempo slower than swimming tempo will not transfer to faster speed in the water.

Finally, at the stage of a swimmer's career when he is specializing in particular events, it is important to focus on strength work that will benefit the swimmer's specialty. Strength work for these specialists should maximize the strong aspects of the swimmer's event and build up the weak points. For instance, if a swimmer is specializing in the 200 fly and has awesome stroke efficiency, but tends to lose tempo on the last 50, the emphasis of strength work should be on training for force (the strong point) as well as building power (the weak point). However, a 50 freestyle specialist who is an awesome finisher but needs to improve reaction time off the blocks, should focus on training for power (the strong point) as well as building explosiveness (the weak point).

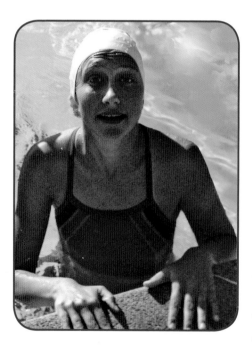

ADAPTATION

Strength training is based on the premise that when muscles are stressed, they adapt to that stress, thus becoming stronger. Because the process of stressing muscles actually creates tiny tears in the muscle fibers, they must be allowed to rest and rebuild before they can become stronger. For this reason, strength building must be considered a long-term activity, designed to build strength gradually over time, using periods of stress and rest.

When adaptation is allowed to occur in this way, it is important that the program evolve, providing new challenges to swimmers as they adapt. Such challenges can take the form of doing the same exercise with more load, more repetitions, or faster repetitions depending on the objective. Or a swimmer could be asked to perform a more complex action than before. Simply repeating the same stress that the swimmer has already adapted to will not increase strength. Each time a swimmer adapts, new demands must be introduced. By using this kind of progression, a swimmer will develop strength more steadily through his or her career.

There is no hard and fast timeline for adaptation. Just as with swimming, strength training does not produce immediate results. Patience is required. A conservative approach, using periodic test sets once a month to gauge adaptation, should determine when new challenges should be presented.

ORIENTATION

When exposed to resistance, muscle fibers adapt and develop, resulting in more strength. The kind of muscle fiber we develop depends on the amount, duration and rate of the resistance. Strength training can develop either slow or fast twitch muscle fiber. Slow twitch muscle fiber is associated with endurance and stamina. Strength training that focuses on developing power builds slow twitch muscle. Slow twitch muscle fiber enables us to do continuous or repetitive movements over a period of time. Fast twitch muscle fiber is associated with speed and agility. Strength training that focuses on developing force and explosiveness builds fast twitch muscle. Fast twitch muscle fiber enables us to sprint and produce bursts of acceleration.

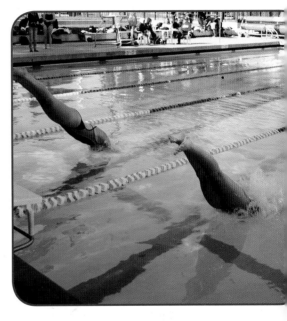

That being said, it is important to remember that in swimming, every event (no matter how short or how long) benefits from both slow and fast twitch muscle strength. While fast twitch muscle fiber is most important for sprinting, even the shortest swimming event requires a number of repetitions of a stroke to be performed over time. Therefore, some slow twitch fiber is also important for the sprinter to have a strong finish. Likewise, while slow twitch is most important for long distance swimming, some fast twitch muscle is essential for the distance swimmer to develop the force and explosive strength that would allow him or her to do quicker starts and all those turns.

Swimming is an activity that builds slow twitch muscle very well. However, not a great deal of fast twitch muscle is built by swimming. This leads some to conclude that the orientation of a strength training program for swimmers should focus on slow twitch development because it is the kind of strength that swimmers use most. But that is only half of the picture. The reason swimmers engage in land-based strength training is to build more strength than they can achieve in the water. If the goal of strength training is more speed then our efforts should address building fast twitch muscle fiber, the type of muscle fiber associated with speed. The most effective strength training program, oriented toward the goal of more speed, must actively address fast twitch muscle development in addition to supplementing the slow twitch work we already get in the pool and need to swim stroke after stroke.

Every individual naturally possesses either more slow twitch muscle or more fast twitch muscle that helps determine what activities they will favor. In swimming, those with more natural slow twitch muscle tend to excel in long distance events and seem to prefer them, while those with more natural fast twitch muscle tend to excel in the sprint events and seem to like them more.

Training, however, can change this. While people are born with a predisposition for endurance or speed, the amount of total muscle fiber responsible for natural ability is very small. In fact, the majority of muscle fiber in the human body is neither fast nor slow twitch. It is convertible, or responsive, to training. Convertible muscle fiber can be trained to work as fast twitch or slow twitch.

This wealth of convertible muscle fiber suggests some interesting possibilities. Would a natural sprinter be able to develop more slow twitch muscle fiber and excel at long distances as well? Would a natural distance swimmer be able to develop more fast twitch muscle and also excel at the sprint events? Certainly the presence of convertible muscle fiber offers swimmers the opportunity to train for more versatility. However, at some point in a swimmer's career, success in certain events leads that swimmer to narrow his or her focus a bit. At that point, training too should be focused toward particular specialties. Training equally for all distances could reduce the results at either extreme. Some sprinters can develop a great deal of bulk, resulting in more resistance and density in the water, in addition to less flexibility that would hinder long distance performance. Conversely, the stroke tempo of most distance swimmers is too slow to achieve great sprinting success. By training for all distances, a swimmer could expect to become pretty fast across the board, but not very fast at any one event. By specializing, a swimmer maximizes performance by training convertible muscle fiber to enhance natural skills.

VARIATION

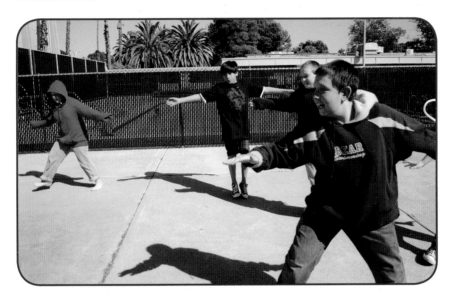

The concept of alternating stress and rest suggests that a swimmer should not do strength training on a daily basis. Actually, for some swimmers, a well-designed strength training program can be done on sequential days, although it is advisable to incorporate one to two days off per week for "pure" rest. The design of a successful daily program accomplishes the stress and rest model by having the swimmer perform upper body exercises on one day and lower body exercises the next day. On the upper body work day, the lower body rests, and on the lower body work day, the upper body rests.

Building in variation in training also keeps a swimmer sharp, both mentally and physically. A creatively designed program uses a diverse array of exercises to meet each training objective. For instance, if the objective is explosiveness, a swimmer could be given leaps for height, 15-yard running sprints, or a speed jump rope activity. If the objective is core stability, a swimmer could be given a two-minute plank, a series of "V" ups, or some "left rights" with a medicine ball. If the objective is power, a swimmer could be given fifteen minutes of rowing, some stretch cord work, or as many dips as they can do in a minute. This sort of variation in training adds interest and can boost a swimmer's coordination, as he or she is required to accomplish new and different actions with the same muscles groups. The crucial point is that every exercise that is added to the mix must bring the swimmer closer to the objective.

Variation also makes things fun. Swimmers spend a lot of time with their faces in the water, alone with their thoughts, looking at the black line on the bottom of the pool. A good variety of land-based strength training gives swimmers the opportunity to socialize while they train, laugh together as they observe each other's initially awkward efforts, and motivate each other as they master the coordination of a new exercise.

OVER-TRAINING

In general, swimmers have a great work ethic. The combination of mental toughness and a highly developed fitness level enables them to keep working when they are tired. While, in many ways, this is an admirable trait, it also leaves swimmers vulnerable to over-training. The danger of over-training becomes a real concern especially when strength training is added to a swimmer's routine. It is important to remember that the main objective of strength training is to enable a swimmer to produce more speed in the pool. If strength training is leaving a swimmer continually too tired to swim well, he or she is probably over-training.

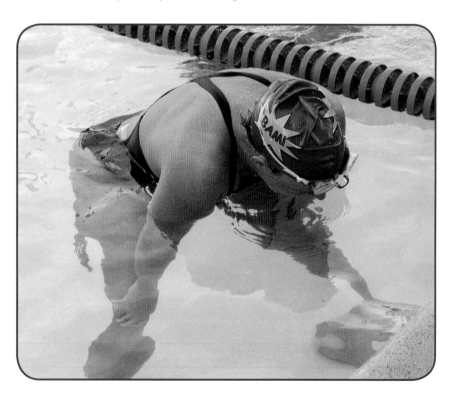

Signs of over-training include continual early fatigue in swim practice, slow tempo, poor race results, plateau, slow adaptation, insomnia, impatience, prolonged grumpiness and lack of interest.

Over-training should be distinguished from the temporary fatigue associated with an intense cycle of training that is followed by a planned cycle of rest, although it may be hard to tell the difference. However, a swimmer who is temporarily fatigued will respond positively to rest and perform better after resting. A swimmer who is over-trained will not show much speed improvement after rest because he has not successfully adapted along the way.

The best way to deal with over-training is to make sure it doesn't happen. Careful and ongoing monitoring of progress is required. This is the responsibility of the coach because often the swimmer will just keep working, focused on the motto he or she has heard throughout his or her swimming career, "If you want to be fast, you have to work hard."

If a swimmer is showing signs of over-training, it should not be ignored. Reduce training, either in terms of duration, intensity or frequency, both in and out of the pool. It might be necessary for the swimmer to take a few days off to recover, then start fresh with a new training plan. If caught early, a few days off will allow a swimmer to get back on the right track. Long-term over-training can result in a season of frustration and an associated drop in confidence and a loss of motivation to continue in the sport.

Coaches must learn to emphasize the fact that rest is good just as strongly as they emphasize the benefits of hard work. The former is a difficult concept for many swimmers to accept, but it is an important one. Sometimes, just working hard does not result in speed; it results in an overly tired swimmer. There is a very fine line between working very hard and working too hard, and every swimmer's threshold is slightly different. Finding each swimmer's balance point is a crucial part of designing a training program that results in faster swimming.

SEASON PLANNING

The goal of strength training is to progressively produce more swimming speed over a swimmer's career, by season, and from meet to meet. Because the ultimate test of the effectiveness of a strength training program is race performance, we must plan our program with competition dates in mind. To ensure that a swimmer is ready to race well, the training plan must accommodate some degree of rest before race day. However, with swim meets scheduled an average of once per week during high school and college seasons, and once every two weeks for age group swimmers, planning for competitions poses training continuity problems. In addition, when frequently accommodating rest before swim meets, the cumulative effect of training is hard to achieve.

For this reason, it is a good idea to look at the season as a whole and work toward a positive conclusion, allowing for benchmark or qualifying opportunities along the way. By defining three levels of competitions, some meets will be identified as priority events and incorporate planned breaks in training, while some will be treated as part of the training.

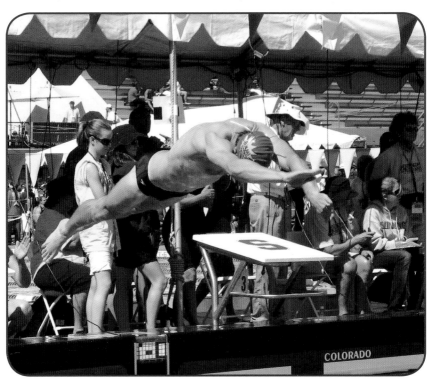

PRACTICE MEETS

In preparation for practice meets, little or no change in the training routine should be made. Just as we "swim through" some competitions, we can also strength train through them. No best times should be expected. Rather than best times, the objective should be stroke quality.

TARGET MEETS

In advance of target meets, the swimmer should be allowed some time to rest. While some swimmers require more rest than others, even one or two days break from the strength training routine can give a swimmer's muscles an opportunity to recover enough to perform well without seriously interrupting the long-term strength training plan. Signs of improvement toward the strength training objective should be visible. Some best times can be expected.

CHAMPIONSHIP MEETS

Strength training should stop about two weeks before the championship meet to allow the swimmer time to adapt and rebuild fully. Although some swimmers get nervous that they will lose their strength, they should be assured that the work they have done on land will be maintained by using it in the pool during this strength training break. Best times should be achieved.

After the competition season, the off-season period can provide a good block of time to build a solid base of well-rounded strength for the next competition season. It also provides the opportunity to make modifications in a swimmer's strength training routine as determined through observation and evaluation of the swimmer's overall performance during the season past.

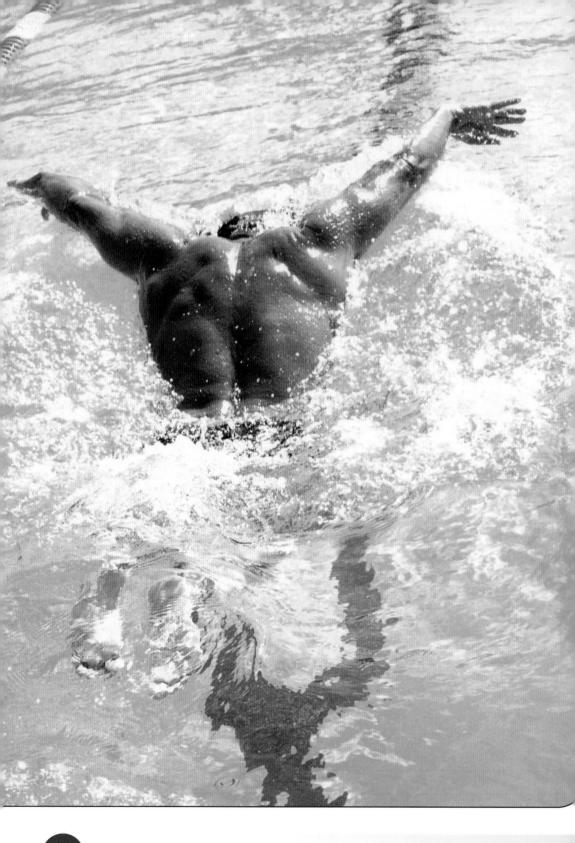

3 THE SWIMMING MUSCLES

Swimming is considered by many to be the best form of full body exercise. The well-documented cardiovascular benefits of swimming focus largely on its healthy effect on the heart and lungs. Upon closer examination, we see that the function of the heart and lungs is to carry oxygen-rich blood to the working muscles and to transport oxygen-depleted blood away from them. What makes swimming particularly good for the heart and lungs is that so many muscles are being used at the same time.

In fact, swimming uses almost every muscle in the body in a coordinated and repetitive, cycling manner that exposes them to sustained exertion in a medium that is thicker than air. Well-conditioned swimmers, in general, have extremely low resting heart rates, a measure of good fitness, and are known to have one of the most developed capillary systems of all athletes. As a swimmer is able to swim farther and faster, the oxygen demand of the muscles increases. As the heart and lungs adapt to meet the demand, new capillaries form, branching out from the existing blood supply network to better provide the muscles in use with more oxygen.

Not only does swimming use more muscles at once than most other sports, it also uses muscles in ways that we don't often use them for other activities. As erect beings, humans spend most of their time using our muscles from the vertical position. However, because swimming is done from a horizontal position, muscle exertion is initiated and carried out in different planes than we are used to. To illustrate this point, compare the actions

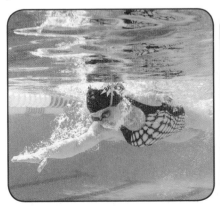 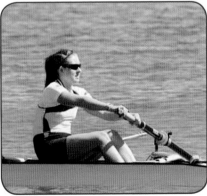

performed with the arms in rowing with those used in swimming. They have many similarities and use many of the same muscles. Rowing, in fact, is a land exercise often recommended for swimmers. Both rowers and swimmers initiate the arm movement with their arms extended in front of them. Both pull toward the body. Both use a cycling arm action. However, in rowing, the athlete's body position is perpendicular to the arms. In swimming, the body is positioned parallel to the arms. This fundamental difference distinguishes the way the muscles exert themselves in swimming from the way they do in rowing and most other land activities.

The foot position of swimmers is another good example of the unique way muscles are used in swimming. Without the ground as a foundation, the feet take on a completely different role in the water. The primary human foot position is perpendicular to the leg, creating a base to stand on and spring from. In swimming, this foot position is used only in a limited fashion for the breaststroke kick, and for starts and turns. Instead, the primary foot position for swimmers is pointed, heel to toe. From this position, it is the top of the foot that applies the most resistance rather than the sole of the feet. This seemingly minor difference is central to how the muscles in the entire leg are used. In fact, it is common for people who are not used to swimming to experience cramps in the calf and in the arch of the foot when they swim due to the different requirements of the muscles when resistance is applied with the top of the foot.

With all this in mind, a strength training program that will be effective for swimmers must consider the full body requirements of swimming, the unique ways swimmers use their muscles, and role each muscle group performs in the act of swimming.

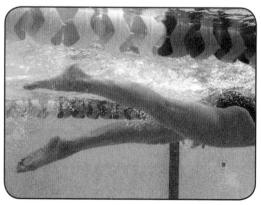 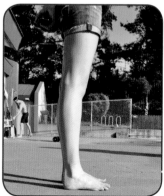

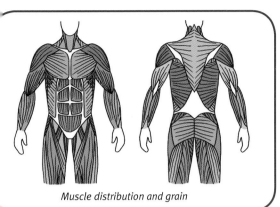

Muscle distribution and grain

LINKING MUSCLE MOVEMENT

Looking at the anatomy of the human body and the distribution of muscles, we can see that the largest muscles are situated closer to the center of the body. We can also see that the fibers that make up each muscle have a distinct grain. By examining the direction of this grain, as well as how the muscles overlap each other, and the point each muscle anchors to the bone, we get an indication of what sort of action each muscle group is capable of and responsible for. With this knowledge, we can better connect muscles to movement and employ them to better move us through the water.

The sequence of muscles called to action in coordinated swimming works in a chain reaction to move the swimmer forward. This flow of energy travels through the body, passing from one muscle group to another throughout each stroke cycle, producing efficient forward motion. Often referred to as the kinetic chain, this connected movement is what a swimmer should strive to simulate in strength training. Rather than isolating one muscle, consider that that muscle is just part of a larger movement.

Imagine a baseball player standing at bat. His arms support the bat, but when he swings to hit the ball, not only will the muscles of his arms come into play but he will employ the muscles in his shoulders, chest, abdomen,

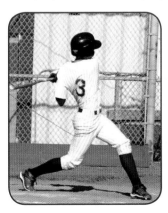

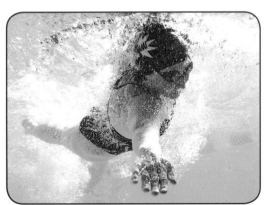

upper and lower back, and legs in one connected motion to send the ball flying fast and far. If instead he used the muscles in his arms in isolation, even with all his strength, the velocity and trajectory of the ball would land it at the pitcher's feet.

It is the same with swimming. An effective swimmer throws his or her body into each stroke, employing not only the muscles of the arms but those in the shoulders, chest, abdomen, upper and lower back, and legs to produce a connected motion with each stroke that moves the body farther and faster, and with less fatigue, than if the arms were used in isolation. An ineffective swimmer moves his or her arms and legs independently of each other, expending a great deal of effort to basically perform four separate actions, rather than one connected action. Linking the muscles together in coordinated movement allows the swimmer to produce better forward motion with less effort.

For this reason, strength training for swimmers should involve multiple muscle groups, to simulate swimming motion as much as possible, rather than training muscles in isolation.

MOVING AND STABILIZING

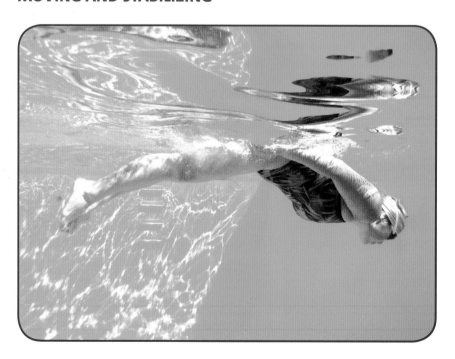

Muscles throughout the body are involved in creating forward movement for the swimmer. Each of these muscles is dedicated to produce specific motions that contribute to the swimming motion as a whole. While muscles create movement for the swimmer, they also have another important function. Muscles also perform as stabilizers. Like in other sports, muscles provide stability to the body in motion and the joints. The muscles that stabilize the knee, for example, keep the bones of the upper and lower leg aligned. Imagine what would happen if there were no stabilizers at the knee; walking, standing, and kicking would be impossible.

Unique to swimming is the additional role of the muscles in providing stability to the moving body as it floats. Without the ground to stand on, swimmers must create their own foundation of stability. In order to move forward in swimming, muscles in one area of the body must be engaged in balancing the effect of an action in another part of the body. These stabilizing muscles maintain tension against the resistance that is being applied. Without good tension, the effect that is produced is not forward motion as desired but a fishtailing or bobbing movement.

Muscles are often categorized as movers and stabilizers. While some muscles serve exclusively as stabilizers, many muscles actually perform both functions. It is the larger surface layer muscles of the core and limbs that can act both as both movers and stabilizers as the body goes through the series of stroke actions that make up swimming. There are several examples of this dual function in swimming.

THE TRAPEZIUS

The trapezius muscle is the large muscle of the upper back that connects the neck and the shoulders and the back. The trapezius moves and rotates the shoulders and neck, as well as stabilizes the shoulder blades and upper body. In freestyle, the trapezius is engaged as a primary mover during breathing as the head turns for the inhale, and during recovery, as the arm moves back to the beginning of the stroke. It also serves as a stabilizer assisting the swimmer in maintaining

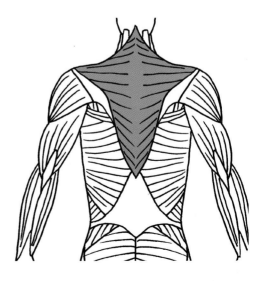

a positive floating position throughout the entire stroke action. When a swimmer presses his or her chest down to achieve the "downhill" floating position, the shoulder blades move closer together. The trapezius is employed in achieving and holding this position.

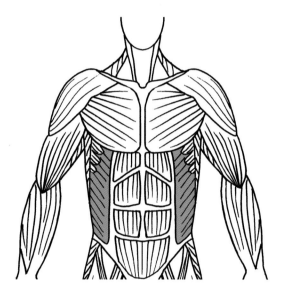

THE OBLIQUES

The obliques are bilateral abdominal muscles located at either side of the "six pack." The function of the obliques is to assist in rotation and sideways stabilization of the body. In freestyle and backstroke, the obliques act in partnership, one as a mover and one as a stabilizer, to produce the pendulum-like roll that provides leverage to the arm stroke. As the swimmer rolls into the stroke, the oblique muscle on the opposite side acts as the primary moving muscle, while the oblique on the same side works to stabilize the core and hips. As the leading arm changes, so does the function of the obliques.

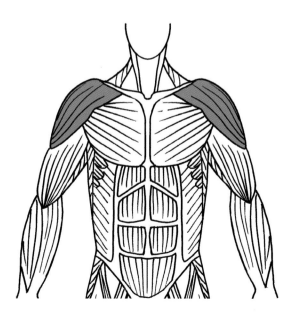

THE DELTOIDS

The deltoids are the bilateral muscles that cover the shoulders. The function of the deltoids is to lift and assist with rotation of the arm. In butterfly, freestyle and backstroke, where the arm recovers out of the water, the deltoids act as primary movers to lift and return the arm to the beginning of the stroke. However, during the power phase of the stroke, the deltoids serve as stabilizers to the shoulder as the arm sweeps through the three-dimensional path of the underwater stroke.

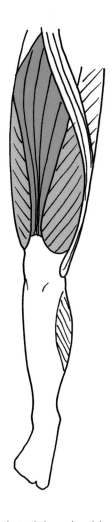

THE QUADRICEPS

The quadriceps are the large and powerful four-part muscles located in the front of the thigh. The function of the quads is to straighten the leg from the hip to the knee and to provide stability to the lower body and knee. In flutter and dolphin kick, the quads are the primary movers as they drive the legs downward for the powerful downbeat of the kick. However, during the upbeat, they serve as knee stabilizers, keeping it from hyper-extending.

Strength training should address both moving and stabilizing. Because the stabilizing effect is more subtle, often strength-building efforts focus on the moving function and ignore the stabilizing function. The importance of self-stabilization in swimming cannot be emphasized enough. We must understand that moving and stabilizing work in partnership. Efficient movement in the water cannot work without both. Therefore strength for moving and strength for stabilizing must be developed in a balanced manner.

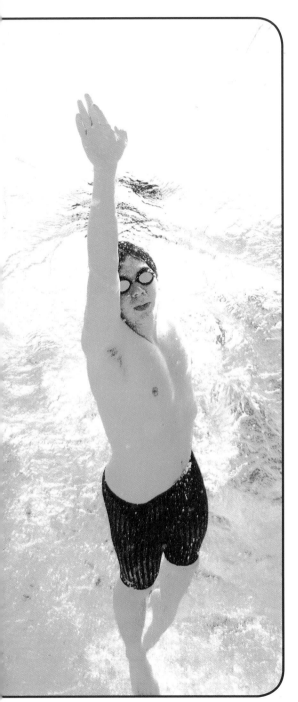

WHAT CONNECTS EVERYTHING

The most obvious muscles used in swimming are in the arms and legs. A quick look at any swimmer in motion shows us that our four limbs are constantly moving. Although it might appear that the arms and legs are our primary movers, in fact, they account for just a small part of a swimmer's propulsion. What connects the four limbs in integrated motion is the core of the body. Like a ceiling fan, with its blades turning, what joins the action of the blades, determines their speed, and generates their power is the motor in the middle.

By generating swimming movements from the motor in the middle – the core –, a swimmer employs the largest muscles to initiate the action and then is able to transfer that motion up to the arms and down to the legs. The relatively smaller muscles of the limbs may ultimately apply the resistance, but the larger muscles of the core are able to produce more force and power, allowing a faster tempo to be created and sustained.

The muscles of the core, both in the front and the back of the body, are also our primary stabilizers. As the connectors between the upper and lower limbs, the tension held in these muscles is central to producing efficient and coordinated stroke action. Without core tension, we would not be able to achieve a unified stroke, produce leverage, or maintain balance and alignment throughout the changing positions of the stroke.

TAKE A SWIMMING LESSON FROM A SEAL

Part of the Pinniped order (from the Latin meaning "wing foot"), we have to look in awe at seals, who are not only among the fastest aquatic mammals but are also the most efficient swimmers. Moving through the water at speeds up to 25 miles per hour (about the same speed as dolphins and whales), seals are at the top of the list in terms of least energy cost associated with producing speed. It seems that seals have perfected swimming.

Like humans, seals are air-breathing mammals, and like us, they have four limbs. However, over millions of years, these descendents of bears have adapted to using aquatic locomotion so well that we should stop and pay attention. Watching the seal swimming at high speed, we see that it holds its front limbs flat against the sides of its body and uses a narrow, undulating motion that starts at the head and moves down through its body.

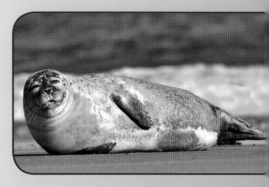

This wave action is based on movement and stabilization of the seal's spine by the muscles that surround it. It is a swimming technique that de-emphasizes the limbs for producing speed in the water. In fact, the seal uses its front limbs for steering rather than propulsion. In addition, the evolution of the seal's rear limbs has led them to be fused into one great limb down to the ankles, creating in essence an extension of the seal's body. By using the muscles of its powerful trunk to produce and control movement, the seal has achieved a "limbless" swimming style that, in comparative studies, has recorded it swimming a distance of one mile more than six times faster than the fastest human swimmer, with five times less effort!

In the absence of evolutionary adaptations such as webbed toes and a streamlined body shape that would make the human form more seal-like, we can learn a lot about swimming from this creature and work toward achieving a more seal-like technique that utilizes the muscles of our core to generate more efficiency and swimming speed.

The muscles of the core are crucial to the overall effectiveness of swimming. Core strength should be a main priority of any strength training program for swimmers. Strengthening the core involves targeting a series of muscles that work together to create a better foundation to swim from. These muscles are listed below.

FRONT CORE MUSCLES

The front core muscles include the abdominals, most visibly the rectus abdominus, commonly known as the "six-pack," which allows forward and backward bending, and provides stability to the core, especially in the horizontal position. Located at either side of the rectus abdominus are the obliques, which assist and stabilize rotation, an important action in long axis strokes. Finally, the major muscles of the chest are the pectoralis major, which are important movers of the arm, especially during the catch and in the beginning of the power phase of all strokes. They also act as stabilizers to the shoulders. Just below the pectoralis major are the serratus anterior, named for their serrated appearance as they cover a portion of the first eight ribs. The function of these muscles is to help raise the shoulder blades, and stabilize the frontal and overhead motions that we use in swimming.

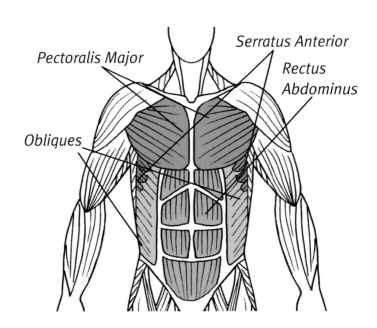

BACK CORE MUSCLES

The largest muscles of the back are the latisimus dorsi, or "lats," which are the primary pulling muscles and are highly developed by swimming. The lats run bilaterally over the length of the back, from under each arm to the waist, and wrap around the swimmer's sides. The trapezius muscle connects the neck to the shoulders and back. It enables a variety of movements including raising and lowering the arm, rotation, turning the head and lifting the shoulders, as well as stabilizing these actions. This is a crucial muscle to maintain as it affects posture and shoulder position. The rhomboids, which are located in the upper back underneath the trapezius, assist in pulling and posture by moving the shoulder blades closer together. Also under the surface layer of muscles in the upper back are the teres major and teres minor muscles. Teres major assists in pulling the shoulders back and rotating the arms outwardly. Teres minor are part of a group of shoulder stabilizing muscles called the rotator cuff. They stabilize internal rotation of the arm.

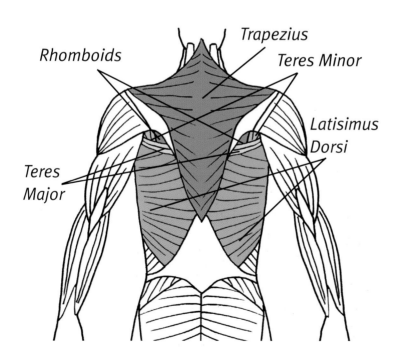

Trapezius

Rhomboids

Teres Minor

Latisimus Dorsi

Teres Major

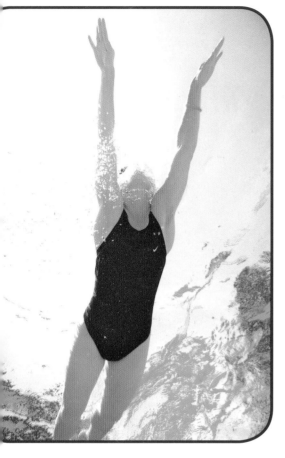

UNDER THE SURFACE

The human body is wrapped with several layers of muscles. It is tempting to target solely the muscles we see, and while these surface-layer muscles are key to producing forward motion in swimming, what lies underneath them is equally important. The function of the underlying muscles is largely to provide stability to the bones at the joints.

In swimming, the joints that get the most use are located in the shoulders. In swimming, we reach, extend and align with our shoulders, use them to apply resistance to the water on multiple planes, and we use them to throw our arms forward to do it all over again. While the extraordinary shoulder enables all of these motions, swimming puts a lot of demand on them. Therefore, taking care of our shoulders should be a priority. Just like a race car designed to perform, to ensure that it is ready to work at an optimal level, regular maintenance of its systems is key. Likewise, our shoulders are so crucial to swimming that maintaining them is just as important. We must both understand their parts and attend to their mechanisms. Shoulder maintenance should be considered a regular part of a strength training program. We must strengthen them from the inside out.

The shoulder has two joints. The first, commonly known as the shoulder joint, lies under the visible deltoid muscle. This joint allows the extensive rotation of the arm that is so basic to swimming. It is a ball and socket type joint, located where the top of the arm bone meets the shoulder blade. Resembling a golf tee, the end of the arm bone sits on top of a shallow socket in the shoulder blade. The remarkable range of motion allowed by this joint ironically makes it vulnerable to instability. The "ball" is held in place on the "tee" directly by four small muscles that surround the joint, stabilizing it during motion. These muscles together are called the rotator cuff.

ROTATOR CUFF

The four muscles of the rotator cuff each have different functions:

Supraspinatus — stabilizes movement of the arm up and away from the body
Subscapularis — stabilizes internal arm rotation
Infraspinatus — stabilizes external arm rotation
Teres minor — stabilizes internal arm rotation and lifting of the arm

When one or more of the rotator cuff muscles is weak, damaged, or develops unevenly, the bones are not held stable and can move around in the joint, leading to inflammation of the surrounding tissues and shoulder pain. In swimmers, poor stroke technique, overuse, or other muscular imbalances can all contribute to rotator cuff problems. But even when these factors are identified and corrected, it is necessary to strengthen the rotator cuff muscles before the shoulder joint can regain stability and perform correctly.

SCAPULAE REGION

The second joint of the shoulder is located at the intersection of the clavicle, commonly known as the collarbone, and the top of the scapulae, commonly known as the shoulder blade. This joint performs like a hinge for the shoulder blade.

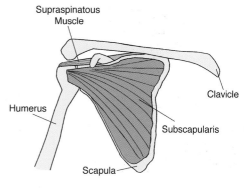

FRONT VIEW

The shoulder blade enables the overhead motions we use in every swimming stroke. Like the shoulder joint, the job of the shoulder blade is to allow extensive motion. To facilitate this, it is held in place only by the muscles, in contrast to most other joints in the body, which also have tendons and ligaments to support them.

When a swimmer has poor posture, weak back muscles or overly developed chest muscles, the shoulder blades can move out of place. The unstable shoulder blade slides upward, tipping out from the back at the lower edge of the bone and tipping into the adjacent structures at the top of the bone. In some swimmers, this condition is visible when looking at the back.

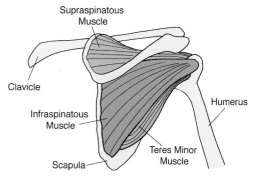

BACK VIEW

One or both of the shoulder blades stick out, away from the body (like wings) and appear to be higher that usual. When the joint continues to do its job, including repeated swimming motions from this wrong position, it can affect the rotator cuff muscles, causing pain. While the rotator cuff is the site of the pain, the cause is instability of the shoulder blade. Although most swimmers with shoulder pain are diagnosed with rotator cuff problems, many physical therapists agree that the primary and underlying cause of all shoulder problems in swimmers is instability of the shoulder blade. Ongoing work to strengthen the muscles that stabilize the shoulder blade should therefore be a priority.

By strengthening the stabilizing muscles that support both shoulder joints, a swimmer can prevent the most common swimming-related health problems. If a swimmer's shoulder does become painful, rest, as well as targeted strengthening exercises of the shoulder stabilizers, should be part of the recovery process.

KEY MUSCLES FOR CERTAIN STROKES

We want to think in terms of multi-muscle swimming movements as much as possible, however because the pull pattern, kicking action, leverage and balance requirements in each of the four competitive swimming strokes is unique, we must consider which muscles are especially important to each stroke.

BUTTERFLY

The wide bilateral recovery of the butterfly places a demand on the trapezius unlike any other stroke. In addition, the initial movements of the power phase are done when the swimmer's body is lower than the chest, requiring the pectoralis 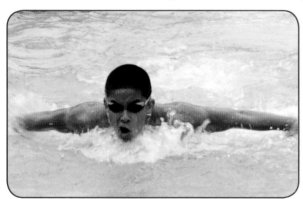 major to engage in a distinct lifting action. Finally, as the dolphin kick places the hips in a higher position relative to the body than in other strokes, the gluteus maximus comes into play.

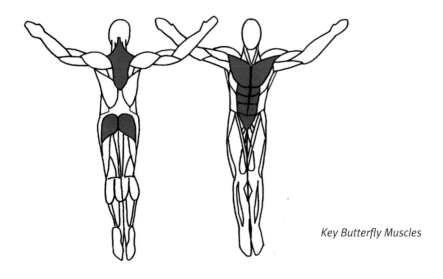

Key Butterfly Muscles

BACKSTROKE

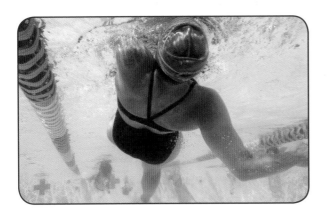

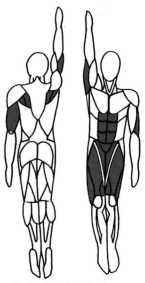

Key Backstroke Muscles

To achieve the ideal body position in backstroke, the pelvis must be tilted forward through abdominal contraction of the retus abdominus. The upward kick, against gravity also puts a large demand on the quads. The unique catch position, behind the head requires the rhomboids to contract heavily. Finally, the elongated push portion of the arm stroke engages the triceps more completely, and for a longer duration than in other strokes.

BREASTSTROKE

The unique requirements of the breaststroke kick engage several muscles that are not otherwise used much in swimming. While the hamstrings are used to raise the heels, the hip flexors and abductors perform and stabilize the sweeping motion of the kick. As the foot position goes from completely feet flexed to completely pointed, the calf muscles are also heavily engaged. The abbreviated breaststroke arm stroke employs the biceps more so than the other strokes during the in-sweep of the

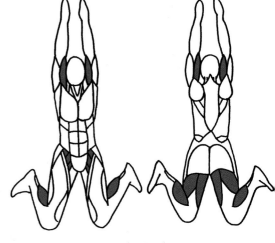

Key Breaststroke Muscles

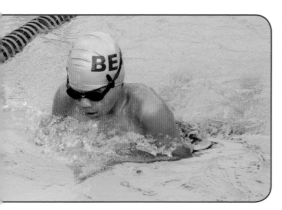

stroke. Finally, the breaststroke's underwater recovery employs the upper trapezius to shrug and roll the shoulders forward as the arms return to the extended position.

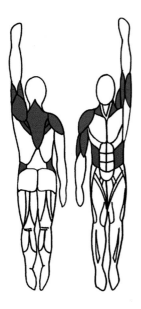

Key Freestyle Muscles

FREESTYLE

The three-dimensional sweeping pull pattern of the freestyle taxes the shoulders more than any other stroke. Rotator cuff muscles and muscles of the scapular region work overtime to stabilize the shoulders in freestyle, as the arms rotate from a high elbow position to the rear of the body during recovery to an extended position in front of the body during the power phase. Finally, the obliques serve as primary movers in freestyle to produce the corkscrew effect that sends power from the core to the upper and lower limbs.

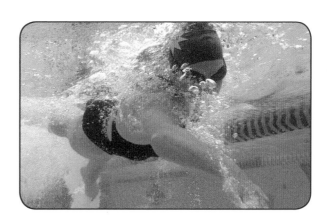

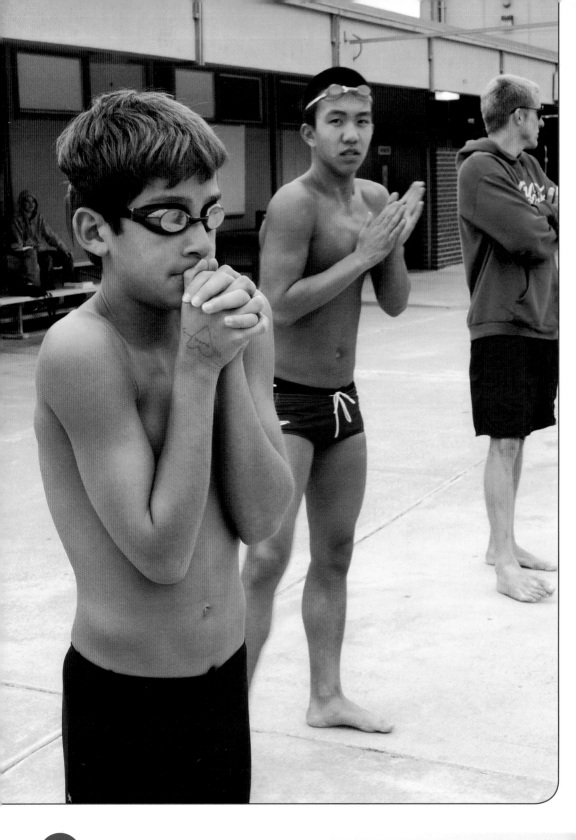

4 STAGES OF DEVELOPMENT AND STRENGTH TRAINING

WHY THIS IS IMPORTANT

Physical development is a process that happens over years. It involves the growth and maturing of every body system. It happens in its own time. Although we may contribute to physical development through good nutrition and healthy living, and we may even exert some control on heightening performance through training, we cannot hurry the actual process of development. While some have tried to influence this process with growth hormones and other drugs, the rewards are very short-lived, and the consequences are great and enduring as the body rebels by becoming sick, injured or shutting down, unable to support artificially accelerated development. Gradual, natural development allows the systems of the body to physically support each other as they grow. The skeleton of a child cannot support the muscles of an adult, but as the child's bones grow, larger muscles and more strength are possible. Gradual development also allows time for important connections to be established between the brain and the body. As we develop, our simple actions evolve into more complex actions over time. Initial, awkward movements become coordinated and seamless.

While people develop at different rates, there is a predictable progression of development that occurs in stages over a lifetime. When designing a strength training program, the stage of development is an important consideration. Strength training encompasses a wide variety of activities, which meet a wide variety of objectives. For every stage, there are particular developmental milestones that should correspond to strength training objectives. As the stage of development changes, strength training objectives must change, too. The content of a strength program should complement the swimmer's abilities at their particular stage and not impose demands that the swimmer is not ready for. A strength training program designed with objectives and activities that fit a swimmer's stage of development will encourage faster swimming at each stage of development and over a swimmer's career.

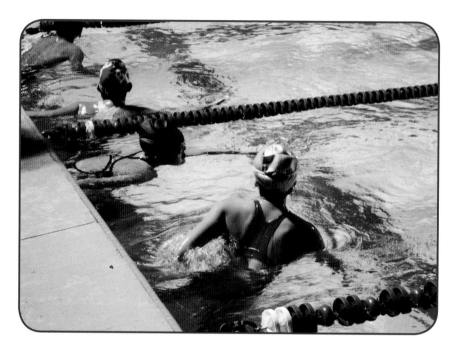

AT WHAT AGE SHOULD STRENGTH TRAINING BEGIN?

The answer to this question is not as simple as how many birthdays a swimmer has had. In fact, there is little benefit to using chronological age as the measure for beginning a strength training program. Chronological age does not tell us much. There are 10-year-olds who are 5'6" and could be mistaken physically for 16-year-olds, and others who are 4'0" tall and could be mistaken for 7-year-olds.

Chronological age also does not address swimming experience. Is the swimmer starting competitive swimming as a teenager, or have they been in the sport consistently since before Kindergarten? Once again, we return to the swimmer's athletic base. A swimmer of any age who does not have an adequate athletic base must be trained as a beginner, although with more physical development, he or she can sometimes advance more quickly than a young beginner.

Rather than chronological age, a more meaningful measure to use is physiological age. Physiological age, or the stage of physical development of a swimmer, provides a better picture of what kind of strength training the swimmer is ready for and can benefit from.

So, at what age should swimmers begin strength training? From day one, but the content of the strength training program must be carefully designed for the appropriate level of physical development and swimming experience.

SPECIFIC WORK FOR SPECIFIC STAGES

We will assign the following categories to the various stages of physical development for the purpose of identifying strength training objective, describing appropriate activities, and suggesting the frequency and duration of strength training sessions. Older beginners should start with the same activities as the first stage listed:

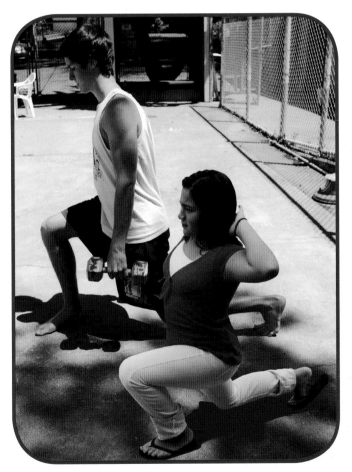

- Elementary
- Pre-adolescence
- Adolescence
- Young Adult
- Adult
- Senior

ELEMENTARY

At this stage, the child's head is proportionally large, and hands and feet are small, leading to some balance issues. The upper body and arm muscles are also generally less developed than lower body and leg muscles. Some children have big bellies, which should be evaluated before labeling the child as overweight. Often a large belly is the result of a growth-related posture imbalance in which the spine curves toward the belly. It is a condition that is usually soon outgrown. Children at this stage have an immense amount of energy but limited coordination and very little endurance.

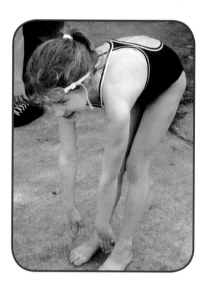

The objective of strength training at this stage of development is to build a solid athletic base. Appropriate strength training sessions three to five days a week, for about 15 minutes, should include activities that promote the five areas of general athleticism – using the child's own resistance only – in short periods of work followed by periods of rest. This work should be fun in order to hold the characteristic short attention span of young children as long as possible.

PRE-ADOLESCENCE

Children at this stage of development experience rapid growth in both height and weight. Often the child has spurts where he or she grows lengthwise and then widthwise, leading to periods of awkwardness. Ultimately, the trunk and limbs lengthen and more strength is possible. Stamina also increases and coordination steadily develops. Balance eventually improves.

The objective of strength training at this stage of development is to improve stability, coordination, and to build

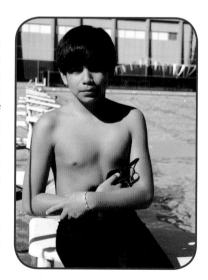

THE EARLY DEVELOPER AND THE LATE BLOOMER

At age 11, Peter was a dedicated member of the swim team who diligently swam five days a week, focusing on good technique and making every interval. He also participated in strength and quickness drills led by his coach three times a week. Peter's work ethic was so admirable that he was given a trophy at the team's annual awards banquet. Peter attended swim meets regularly, holding clearly in his mind the goal of swimming faster than ever before.

One day, after placing fifth in his favorite event, the 50 butterfly, he looked at the field of swimmers at the finish and spotted his teammate Allen raising his fist in victory. "Good for him!" Peter thought momentarily as a sense of confusion welled up inside of him and set in. Allen wasn't a hard worker. He fooled around a lot and snuck out of practice early all the time. How could he have won the race?

Peter's coach approached both his swimmers with enthusiastic congratulations. As they stood side by side, Peter was struck by the fact that his teammate was nearly a head taller than he was. He had never noticed how much Allen had grown or how husky his voice had become. At the end of the meet, he confided in his coach, asking why he wasn't improving like Allen was. His wise coach pointed out that Peter was progressing and, in fact, had done his best time. He said it was important to be patient and keep up his good training. "Your day will come, Peter," the coach told him.

Peter held on to his coach's words. Over the next year and a half, Peter trained regularly, both in and out of the water, developing a well-defined six pack that he was proud of. Eventually, Allen decided to trade in his jammers for a soccer ball. Peter kept whittling away slowly and patiently at his times in competition and, after advancing to the 13-14 division, he adopted the 100 fly as his new favorite.

At the first meet of spring, Peter stepped up on the blocks, seeded tenth in the fly. He swam the first 50 with ease and precision but felt uneasy when he found himself with more energy than usual going in the last lap. Intent on giving the race his best, he put his head down and accelerated his stroke tempo. When the final wall came, Peter looked up and was shocked to see he had won the race, erasing nine full seconds from his previous best time. As he emerged from the pool, he heard a familiar voice. "I told you!" the coach said. Peter grinned widely. It was only then that he observed that he was not looking up at his coach, but looking at him eye to eye. He realized at that moment that his patience had paid off, and it was finally his turn to shine.

power. Appropriate strength training activities for this stage of development include exercises that address core stability balance and tempo, using the child's own resistance only. This is a good stage to start focusing on perfecting form that will carry through to later stages of development. Such work can be done three to four days a week in sessions of about 20 minutes.

ADOLESCENCE

During adolescence, athletes go through a time of continuous change that includes physical maturing and weight gain. As they go through puberty, athletes experience periods of rapid strength gain alternating with periods where strength lags behind their growth. At times, their physical changes are accompanied by awkwardness and self-consciousness. At other times, they are accompanied by bravado and testing of their new characteristics.

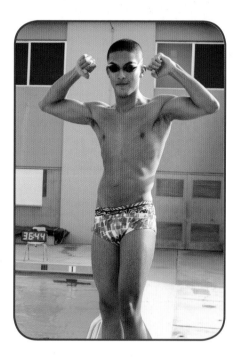

The objective at this stage of development is building power, force, stability, and coordination. When well supervised, swimmers can make important progress during this time, with gains in applicable strength. Sessions of 30 minutes or more, five days a week should include self-resistance work, medicine balls and some stretch bands, accompanied by clearly stated objectives. This combination of training can encourage swimmers to focus on achieving great improvements in swimming speed.

YOUNG ADULT

At this stage, the athlete has adult physical characteristics and size. This is a period when the athlete is at the peak of strength and performance potential. With a solid foundation of athleticism, swimming and strength work, the now fully mature swimmer can make huge and continuing gains in speed with dedication to a solid training routine and a healthy lifestyle.

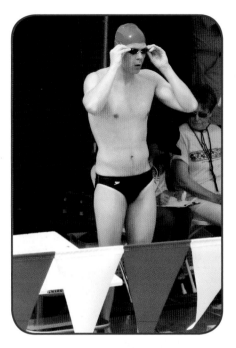

The objective at this stage is maximizing force, power, and explosiveness. A strength program that encompasses weight training, stretch bands, medicine balls and self-resistance can encourage development of maximum strength by the athlete's adult body that can be applied to swimming faster than ever before. A program of strength work four days a week for an hour can net the force, power, explosiveness, and stability results of a lifetime.

ADULT

During this stage, a very gradual decline of muscle size and strength is expected. The shape of the body changes subtly over time, frequently expanding at the waistline. With the obligations of "real life," the adult athlete faces less training time and, in general, a less active lifestyle.

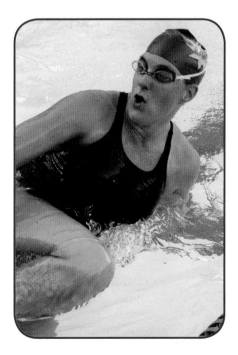

For the adult athlete, the objective is maintenance. Holding on to physical fitness is certainly a challenge. As the years go by, maintenance should be viewed as improvement! With an ongoing routine of frequent swimming and strength work, it is possible for a swimmer to maintain his or her speed into the 40s and 50s.

A routine that includes strength training for an hour encompassing weights, stretch bands, medicine balls and self-resistance for three days a week will provide such maintenance. At this stage, it is important to make time for two days of solid rest as recovery just takes longer.

SENIOR

In the golden years, decline in the size and strength of muscles is evident, which sometimes contributes to balance and mobility problems. In addition, seniors can face bone strength and flexibility issues affecting posture and range of motion. Still, the senior who stays active and strong will be in a much better position to make the most of his or her ability to move freely through the water.

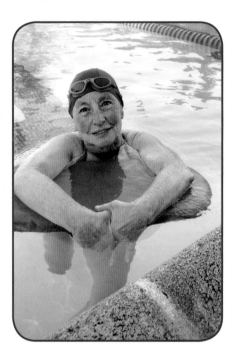

At this stage of development, the objective is flexibility and weight-bearing activity. Strength training is an essential part of a swimmer's training routine. A program that includes conservative weights, stretch cords, and medicine balls, as well as self-resistance, two to three days a week for 30 minutes or more can produce bone density improvements, slow muscle decline, and along with the typical benefits of swimming, contribute to a better quality of life.

JUST KEEP SWIMMING

Joy was a dedicated mother. For almost two decades, she devoted herself to the task of raising her twins to become happy, healthy, productive adults. She parented to encourage individuality, responsibility, compassion and self-respect. She strived to be a good example to her children. On their 18th birthday, Joy felt an immense sense of pride. Still, shortly thereafter, when they moved out on their own, she felt empty inside. A divorced 48-year-old, Joy looked at herself in the mirror and asked, "Who am I?" Her empty house and the new availability of time took quite a while to adjust to, but one day, Joy woke up with an idea.

One of the good examples she had provided for her children was to maintain a regular physical fitness routine throughout their childhood. An active competitive swimmer in her youth, Joy had chosen swimming as her fitness activity, going to the pool twice a week before daylight for an hour or so to swim laps. Although she was no longer a speed demon in the pool, she had maintained a healthy weight, good muscle tone and flexibility that other mothers often admired.

Now that she didn't have to hurry back home to meet the responsibilities of the household, she decided to re-dedicate herself to her sport. She increased her swimming time, adding another day a week, and then another half hour per session. She added variety to her swimming routine by doing sets and different strokes. It was not long before Joy started feeling the effects of her efforts and soon was able to do 100s on the 1:30 like she had when she was a teenager.

Swimming became the passion in Joy's life. She loved the challenge and confidence that swimming gave her. She kept track of her workouts, recording her yardage and tracking her progress toward benchmarks she set for herself. She read books on swimming science and technique, and incorporated what she learned into her swimming routine, even adding some stretch cord work to her program three times a week.

At age 65, Joy was thrilled to become the grandmother of twins. To celebrate this milestone, she decided to enter a competition for adult swimmers. With anticipation, but no expectations, she arrived at the event and was pleased that she, by no means, was the oldest swimmer present. Elated by the camaraderie and positive atmosphere she encountered, she swam to a second place finish in the 200 backstroke. The winner, a woman of at least 80, congratulated her as she climbed easily out of the pool. "Maybe, I'll see you at the next meet," Joy responded. "Yes, you will," the woman asserted. "Until then, just keep swimming."

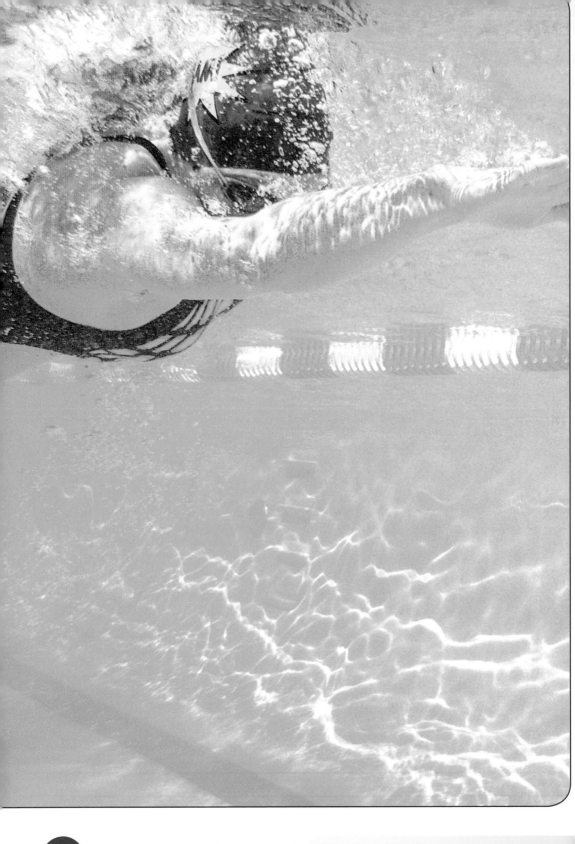

5 LET'S GET SPECIFIC

TYPES OF STRENGTH TRAINING THAT BENEFIT SWIMMING

This section introduces five kinds of strength training that benefit swimming in terms of building strength that is useable in the water. Under each of the five types of activity, specific exercises are listed. Each exercise has been selected for its transferability to swimming in terms of directionality, tempo and multi-muscle engagement. Each exercise is described, illustrated, and categorized by the area of the body it primarily targets. It is important to remember that although an exercise is described as targeting a particular area of the body, multiple muscles are involved, both in the target area, as well as in other areas of the body. For instance, exercises that target the upper body and arms usually involve the core as well.

While all strength training is based on resistance, each type of exercise presented provides a different kind of challenge to the muscles. Some types are appropriate for all swimmers, but some are appropriate only at more advanced stages of development and are noted as such.

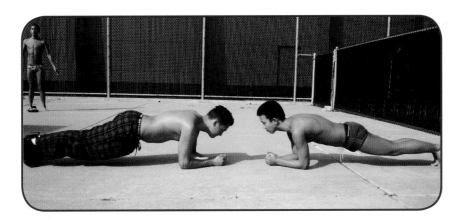

SELF-RESISTANCE

Self-resistance refers to using the weight of one's own body as the load. "Baby stuff!" you might say; far from it. Some of the most beneficial and challenging exercises for swimmers of all levels fall under this category. Self-resistance work, in fact, should be a part of all strength training programs, as it resembles swimming very closely in terms of multi-muscle movements. Self-resistance work promotes core stability and balance, coordination and tempo. In addition, force, power, and explosiveness can all be developed very successfully with self-resistance work.

Beneficial self-resistance activities include:

FULL BODY

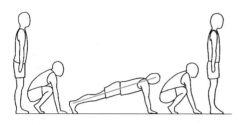

Burpies — Stand, squat, extend legs, squat and stand. Repeat the sequence.

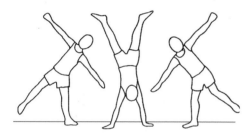

Cartwheels — A gymnastics handspring where the body turns over sideways and back to the standing position with the arm and legs spread like the spokes of a cartwheel.

Crab Walk — Walk on all four limbs with the back toward the ground.

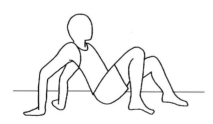

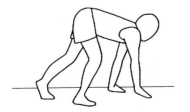

Crawling — Walk on hands and feet.

Speed Walking — As in the Olympic sport, a rapid heel to toe walking stride using leverage from the arms and core.

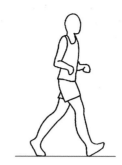

Cherry Pickers — Stand with legs wider than shoulders. Bend down and with both hands, touch left foot with both hands. Then touch the ground between the feet, move to the right foot and then stand up straight. Repeat.

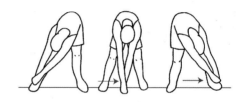

Jumping Jacks — Standing with arms at sides, jump up and clap your hands over your head at the same time as you spread your legs and land in that position. Recover along the same path and repeat in rapid succession.

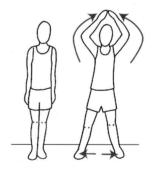

Running — Use swift heel to toe strides on one foot with the opposite side arm bent at the elbow, and move in the same direction simultaneously.

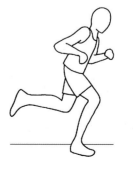

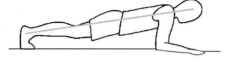

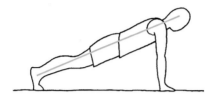

CORE

Plank — Holding the core firm, place yourself face down while supporting the body on the elbows and toes.

Variation: High Plank — Holding the core firm, place yourself face down while supporting the body on the hands and toes, like a high push-up position.

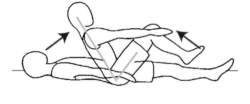

V Ups — Lying on your back, raise the legs and the upper body to the middle at the same time, creating a "V."

Variation: Start with arms extended overhead, and raise the arms and upper body with the leg and feet so the hand and feet touch in a high "V."

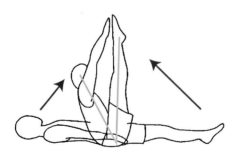

Left, Right, Ups — With knees bent, and hands supporting the back of the neck, do a sequence of crunches to the left, to the right, and straight up, raising the shoulder blades off the ground.

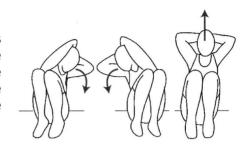

Leg Lifts — Lying on your back, with hands under hips, lift the feet off the ground six inches and hold, then 6 more inches up and hold, then 6 more inches up and hold. Do the reverse back down.

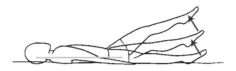

Air Kicking — Lying on your front with arms extended, raise head, with arms and feet about 12 inches off the ground and do a narrow, rapid flutter kick. Variation: Do the same lying on back.

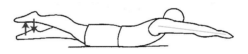

Insect — Lying on your back, with arms extended over the head, lift the shoulders off the ground and bring the left hand and the right foot together in the middle. Then, as they return to the starting position, bring the right hand and left foot together, and repeat rapidly.

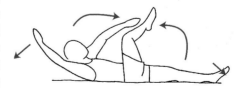

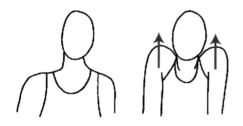

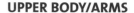

UPPER BODY/ARMS

Shrugs — While standing, lift the shoulders up toward the ears, then release. Repeat.
Variation: Lift the shoulders up and roll them forward or backward.

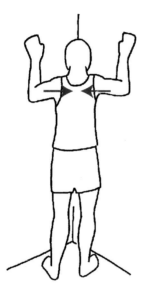

Corner Push Out — Facing a corner, with the hands on the wall at shoulder level and width, bring the chest into the corner, squeezing the shoulder blades together until the elbows are at 90 degrees, then return to the starting position. Repeat.

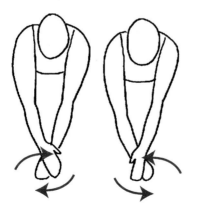

Hand Switch — With arms extended at shoulder height, perpendicular to the body, move the left hand out and over the right hand, then right hand out and over left hand in rapid succession repeatedly.

Quick Clap — With eyes closed and arms at sides, bring the hands together in a clap as quickly as possible when a signal such as a whistle or beep is given. Return arms to sides. Repeat with randomly timed signals to promote quick reaction time.

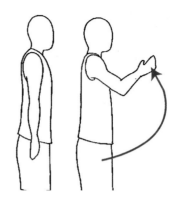

Relaxed Arm Circles — From a standing position, with arms extended from the sides, swing arms in relaxed continuous circles to the front. Repeat circling to the back.

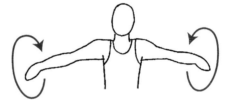

Hanging Arm Circles — Stand with your feet wider than your shoulders, bend over at the waist and allow your left arm to hang down, relaxed. Gently swing your arm in continuous circles to the left. Repeat circling to the right. Perform the exercise again with the other arm.

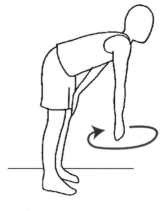

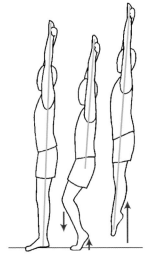

LEGS

Streamlined Leaps — Standing with arms extended over head and squeezing the ears, hand over hand, bend the knees and spring straight up, then land on the balls of the feet, repeatedly. Attempt to land in exactly the same position each time.

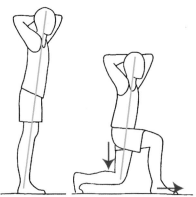

Lunges — Standing with hands clasped behind the head and elbows out to the sides, take a giant step forward, lowering the knee of the back leg almost to the ground. Return to the standing position. Do the same with other leg leading. Repeat.

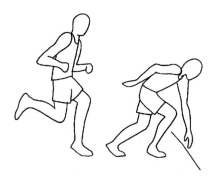

Running Lines — With five lines drawn on the ground about 5 yards apart, run to the first line, touch it and return to the starting point, then run to the second line, touch it and return to the starting point, and continue the pattern through all five lines.

Variation: Build up 1 to 5 lines, and then build down 5 to 1 lines. (Do you mean starting at the farthest line and doing the longer runs down to the shortest?)

Frog Jumps — From a full squat position, explode upward. Repeat a few times.

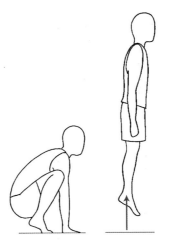

Skipping — Hop forward on one foot and then the other rhythmically and repeatedly.

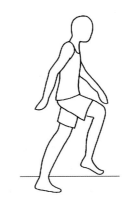

Side Steps — With arms extended out to the sides at shoulder level, take a large stride sideways with the leading leg, then bring the trailing leg to meet it, and repeat in rapid succession. Repeat using the opposite leg to lead.

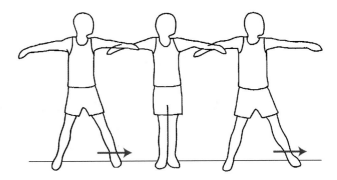

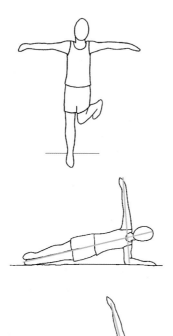

BALANCE

One Leg Balancing — With arms extended to the sides, stand on one foot and hold. Repeat standing on the other foot.
Variation: Maintain balance with arms in various positions.

Side Plank — Beginning in the plank position and holding a firm core while supporting the body face down on the elbows and toes, rotate the body to the side extending the high arm into the air for balance. Hold. Repeat on other side.
Variation: High Side Plank – Beginning in the high plank position and holding a firm core while supporting the body face down on the hands and toes, rotate the body to the side extending the high arm into the air for balance. Hold. Repeat on other side.

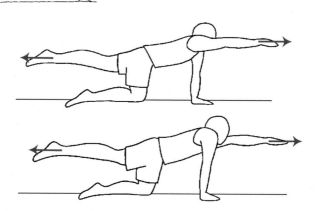

Alternating Extensions — From the face-down position resting on hands and knees, extend the right arm forward and the left leg back in line with the body, hold, then return to the starting position. Do the same with the opposite limbs.

WHERE ARE THE PUSH-UPS?

The traditional push-up, a mainstay of modern exercise and a standard measure of fitness level, does not appear among these recommended self-resistance exercises intentionally. Although countless push-ups are done regularly by pro-athletes, military recruits, and even Rocky, as part of their physical training routines, it is the belief of this coach that the push-up should not be part of a swimming strength training program.

The push-up does not address swimming very well. It does not simulate swimming motion at all, as the direction of the resistance is perpendicular to the athlete's body, rather than parallel. While the push-up does promote core and upper body strength, it also taxes the shoulders in ways that do not benefit swimming. Extensive push-ups can develop muscles that interfere with a swimmer's range of motion in the water, especially during arm extension. Further, the push-up shortens shoulder stabilizers and chest muscles where they already tend to be too short among swimmers.

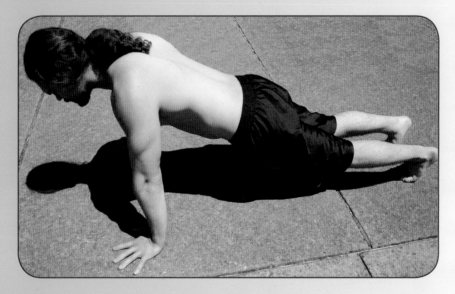

Activities that are less problematic for swimmers, that promote swimming-specific core and upper body strength better than the push-up, include the plank, side plank and corner push out.

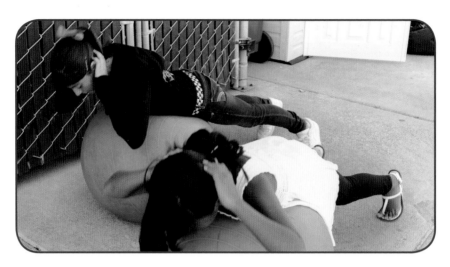

SELF-RESISTANCE WITH ACCESSORIES

Small accessories can be included to add complexity or challenge to self-resistance work. Accessories include balls, jump ropes, hula hoops, cones, rope, and balance balls. Self-resistance work can also take advantage of landscape features, including sand, stairs, bleachers and hills. Playground and gymnastic equipment, including bars, rings, nets and pegboards, may also be used. Close supervision should always be maintained.

Good "accessorized" self-resistance work includes:

FULL BODY

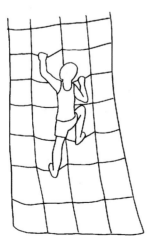

Net Climbing — Use the arms and legs to ascend a net made of rope.

Rope Climbing — Use the arms and legs to ascend a rope.

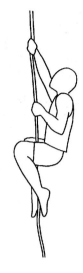

Skating — Move and balance while wearing roller skates, roller blades or ice skates.

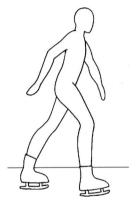

CORE

Hula Hoop — Keep the hula hoop spinning around the waist through rhythmic core movements.

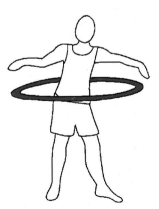

Balance Ball Passes — Lying on back with arms extended over the head, hold the balance ball in your hands. Simultaneously lift your shoulder blades off the ground, bringing the balance ball toward the middle of your body. As you raise your knees and feet to the middle of your body, pass the ball to your feet and return to the starting position, with your feet holding the balance ball. Repeat, passing the balance ball to the hands.

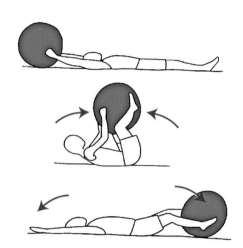

Balance Ball Crunches — Face up, with hips on balance ball, feet on floor, and hands crossing the chest do crunches repeatedly.

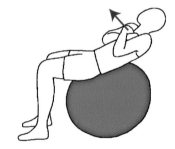

Balance Ball Chest Lifts — Face down, with hips on balance ball, feet on floor, and hands clasped in back of head, raise and lower the chest repeatedly.

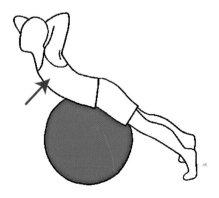

Sky Crunches — Lying down with knees bent and lower legs resting on a chair or bleachers, keep hands and chin pointed to the sky while lifting shoulders off the ground repeatedly

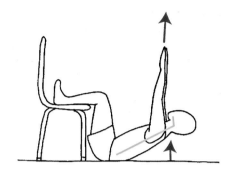

UPPER BODY/ARMS

Body Lifts — Stand facing a bar that is at least shoulder height. Reaching directly up, grasp the bar, palms down with the hands about shoulder width apart. Lift the body up as if you are climbing out of the pool. Return to the starting position and repeat.

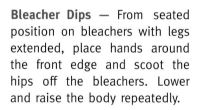

Bleacher Dips — From seated position on bleachers with legs extended, place hands around the front edge and scoot the hips off the bleachers. Lower and raise the body repeatedly.

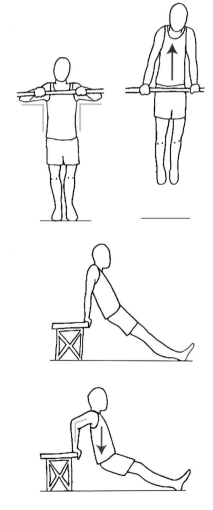

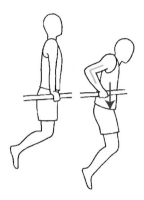

Bar Dips — Hold the body off the ground between parallel bars, and lower and raise the body repeatedly.

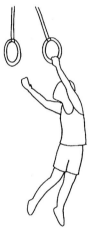

Rings — Using playground or gymnastics rings, swing from ring to ring.

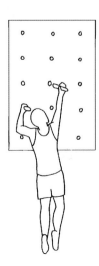

Pegboard — Grip pegs in lower holes of board and hang from pegs. Ascend the board by hanging with one arm while using the other arm to put the peg in a higher hole. Repeat with alternating arms until the top of the board is reached.

LEGS

Stairs — Climb up a long flight of stairs quickly.

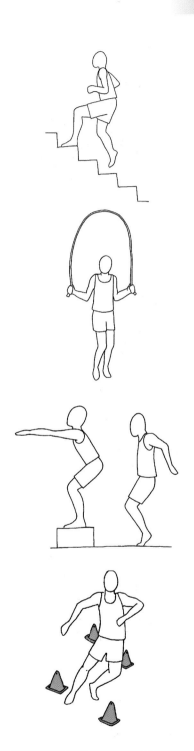

Jump Rope — Holding the ends of a length of rope in each hand, swing it over the head and under the feet repeatedly, jumping over it as it approaches the feet, adding a small rhythmic jump between each jump over the rope.
Variation: Speed Jump Rope — Jumping rope at high speed without the additional small rhythmic jump between each jump over the rope.

Box Jumps — Standing on the ground behind a crate, bend the knees and jump up explosively on to it, and then jump down. Repeat.

Zig Zags — With a line of small cones spaced about 15 inches apart, stand to the right of the cones. Quickly step to the left between the first two cones, then to the right between the second and third cone, then to the left between the third and fourth cone, until every cone has been passed between in a rapid zig-zag pattern.

BALANCE

Balance Ball — Alternating Limb Balance — Lying face down with the trunk on a balance ball and the feet on the ground, raise the right arm and left leg off the ground and hold. Repeat with opposite limbs.

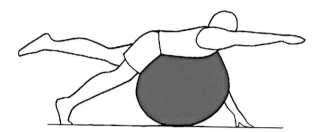

Balance Ball — Single Leg Front — Lying face down with the trunk on the balance ball and arms extended over the head, raise the left leg off the ground in line with the body and hold. Repeat with opposite leg.

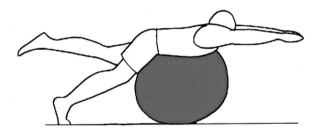

Balance Ball — Single Leg Back — Lying face up with the back on the balance ball and arms extended over the head, raise the left leg off the ground in line with the body and hold. Repeat with opposite leg.

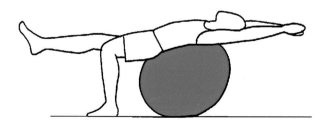

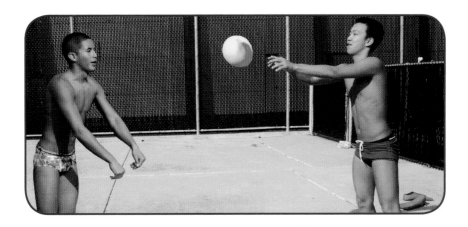

THE MEDICINE BALL

The medicine ball is a weighted ball that can be used to perform a wide variety of strength training work. The medicine ball provides a compact external load in useful weights from 1 to 25 pounds. Even with this minor amount of added resistance, medicine balls are not recommended for swimmers in the earliest stages of development for two reasons. First, they are weights, and the bones of young athletes are not physically ready to support more than their own body weight. Second, although medicine balls may look like toys, and in many ways act like a regular ball (they can be tossed, rolled and caught), they must be handled as tools. They are heavy and, if dropped on a foot or thrown at someone's face, they can cause injury. Medicine balls should be used only by athletes with the maturity to handle them carefully.

There are many benefits of medicine ball training. It allows the swimmer to move through multiple planes, which simulates the movement used in swimming, unlike traditional weightlifting, which is done in a single plane. Medicine ball activities encourage the swimmer to develop both moving and stabilizing functions evenly as he or she must exert effort to move the ball and stabilize to control the ball. Medicine ball training also helps develop force and explosiveness very well, as the swimmer must react quickly to the weight of the ball when it comes toward him and when he sends it into flight. Finally, medicine ball training encourages coordination by using multi-muscle movements rather than isolated muscle efforts.

Medicine balls can be used by an individual and, in some cases, with a partner. Beneficial activities for swimmers include:

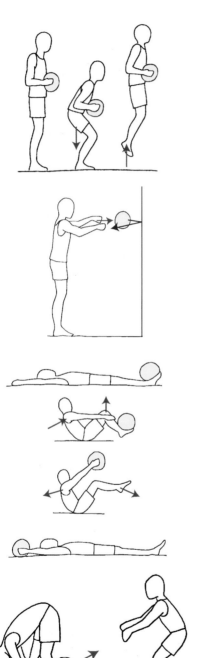

FULL BODY

Squat and Jump — Hold the ball with two hands at about the belly button level, squat, then jump into the air explosively. Repeat.

Standing Wall Rebounds — Stand 3-5 feet away from a wall. Throw the ball forcefully at the wall from chest level. Catch it as it rebounds. Repeat rapidly.

Leg Lift and Pass — Lying on the back with the arms extended over the head and the medicine ball balanced on the tops of the feet, bend the knees and draw the legs toward the middle while bringing the upper body to the middle so that the hands can reach the ball. Take the ball in the hands and return to the starting position. Repeat after placing the medicine ball onto the tops of the feet.

Hike (with partner) — As in football, toss the ball between the legs toward a partner behind you. Switch. Repeat.

CORE

Left, Rights — Seated on the ground and holding the medicine ball at your belly button, lean back and raise the knees, keeping the feet flat on the ground. Rotate your upper body to the left and touch the ground with the medicine ball, then rotate to the right and touch the ground with the medicine ball. Repeat.

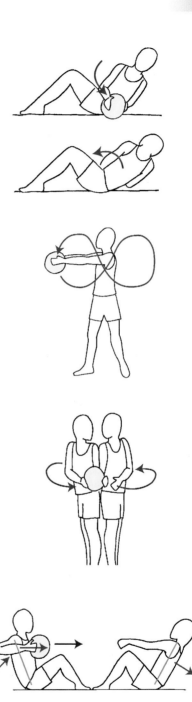

Figure Eights — Standing with legs at least shoulder width apart, hold the medicine ball out from the chest with extended arms. Move the arms in the shape of a figure eight, half to the left of the body and half to the right. Repeat.

Pass Arounds (with partner) — Standing back to back with a partner, rotate the body to the left, without moving the feet and pass the medicine ball to your partner who has rotated her body to receive the ball. Repeat, rotating in the opposite direction. Continue.

Crunch Toss (with partner) — Lying on the back, knees raised, toe to toe with a partner, hold the medicine ball against the chest, lift the upper body off the ground and toss the medicine ball to your partner. As your partner catches the ball, both partners return to the starting position. Repeat rapidly.

UPPER BODY/ARMS

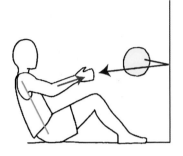

Seated Wall Rebounds — From a sitting position, leaning back with bent knees, about 3-5 feet from a wall, throw the medicine ball forcefully at the wall and catch it as it rebounds. Repeat rapidly.

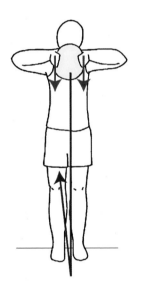

Throwdowns — From a standing position, holding the medicine ball above the head, throw it down to the ground forcefully and catch it as it rebounds. Repeat rapidly.

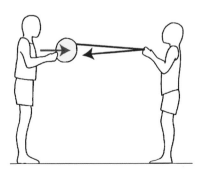

Quick Toss (with partner) — Standing 6-10 feet apart, toss the medicine ball to a partner with two hands. Your partner catches it and, in the same motion, tosses it back. Repeat rapidly.

LEGS

Squats — Holding the medicine ball close to the body at the level of the belly button, squat and stand repeatedly, maintaining posture and balance

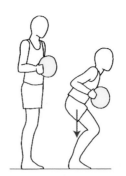

Step Ups — Holding the medicine ball close to the body at the level of the belly button, step up onto a crate or bleacher, then step down. Repeat with opposite leg leading.

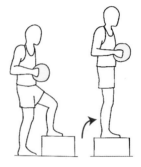

Lunges — Holding the medicine ball close to the body at the level of the belly button, take a large stride forward, allowing the trailing knee to approach the ground. Stand and bring the trailing leg forward. Repeat. Perform the same action with the other leg leading.

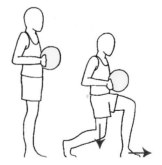

BALANCE

All of the above exercises.

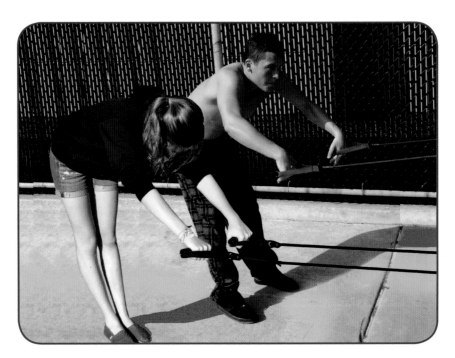

STRETCH CORDS

Without a doubt, stretch cords provide one of the best swimming-specific methods of strength training. Stretch cords are simply lengths of surgical tubing with loops or handles for each hand. When secured in the middle to a stationary pole, the stretch cord enables the swimmer to simulate the entire range of motion that makes up the power phase of the stroke against resistance. Stretch cords also require the use of an accelerating motion to accomplish the action successfully, exactly like swimming. The motion is repeated with a controlled reverse action or recovery between each exertion. The swimmer can use a tempo equal to his or her swimming tempo against resistance or practice an "ideal" higher tempo. Stretch cords also promote core stabilization, as the swimmer must maintain constant tension in the body from the standing position, bent forward at the waist, while the arms are moving.

Stretch cords are available in a variety of thicknesses, which determine their resistance. Because too much resistance will make proper technique impossible, it is important to start with a stretch band that has less resistance and work up to more resistance when good technique is maintained.

The following stretch cord exercises are highly recommended:

FULL BODY

Double Arm Pull — Standing and bent forward at the waist, hold the stretch cord in both hands and perform the underwater path of butterfly, accelerating throughout. Recover gently following the same path. Repeat.

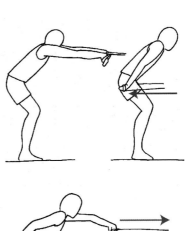

Alternating Arm Pull — Standing and bent forward at the waist, hold the stretch cord with both hands and perform the underwater path of freestyle, accelerating toward the end with one arm while the other recovers gently following the reverse path. Repeat in an alternating manner.

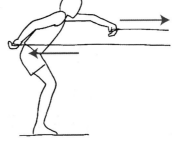

Double Triceps Press — Standing straight, hold the stretch cord with both hands, with the elbows at a right angle and firmly against the sides of the body. Straighten the arms quickly without moving elbows. Recover gently along the same path. Repeat.

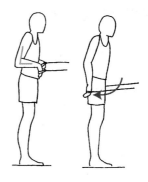

Alternating Triceps Press — Standing straight, hold the stretch cord with both hands, with elbows at a right angle and firmly against the sides of the body. Straighten one arm quickly without moving the elbow, then reverse the motion as the other arm straightens quickly without moving the elbow. Repeat in an alternating manner.

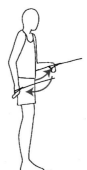

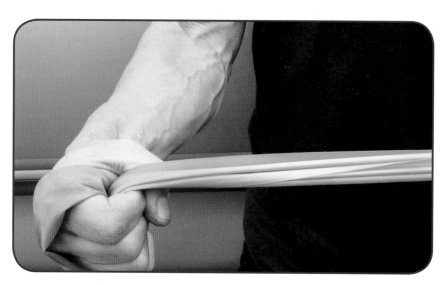

STRETCH BANDS

Closely related to the stretch cord is the stretch band. The stretch band is an excellent tool for shoulder maintenance. Also known as a therapy band, this narrow sheet of latex provides much less resistance than the stretch cord, which is not recommended for shoulder stabilization work.

Stretch band exercises for shoulder stability include:

UPPER BODY/ARMS

External Sweep — With one end of the stretch band anchored at elbow level to the left of the body, hold the other end of the band in the right hand,

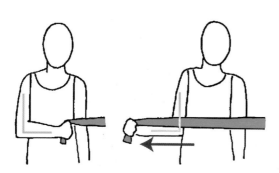

across the belly button, with the elbow bent to 90 degrees and held firm to the side of the body. Swing the lower arm outward as if it were a door opening. Recover along the same path. Open and close repeatedly. Anchor stretch band to the right of the body and repeat motion with right arm.

Internal Sweep — With one end of the stretch band anchored at the elbow level to the left of the body, hold the other end of the band in the left hand outside the body, with the elbow bent to 90 degrees and held firm to the side of the body. Swing the lower arm inward as if it were a door closing. Recover along the same path. Close and open repeatedly. Anchor stretch band to the right of the body and repeat motion with the right arm.

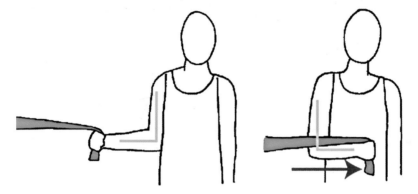

Back Scrubber — With the length of the stretch band folded in half, hold one end of the stretch band in the left hand and raise the hand over your head, palm back, then drop the elbow down so the stretch band dangles down the back. With the right hand, reach down behind the back and grasp the other end of the stretch band. Gently pull the band up with the left hand, then down with the right hand repeatedly, as if scrubbing the back. Repeat with hands in opposite positions.

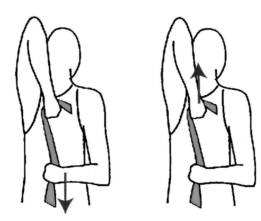

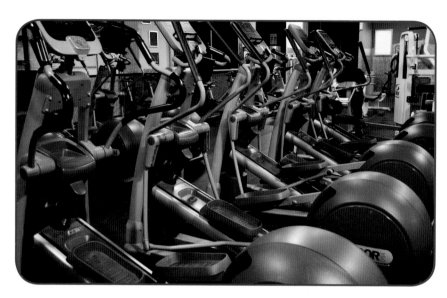

EXERCISE MACHINES

Exercise machines provide a great aerobic component to a land-based routine, raising the heart rate and contributing to endurance. Many are valuable for developed athletes as a warm-up before lifting weights or performing other strength training activities. A few contribute additional opportunities for building force and explosiveness as well. As they are designed for adult frames, they should not be used by young children.

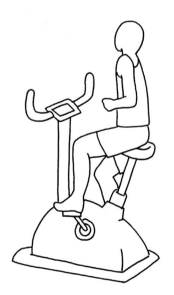

The best exercise machines for warm-ups are listed below:

Exercise Bike — A stationary bicycle that can be set at various resistances. Comes in reclining or upright models. Either model is good, but with the upright model, use without holding handlebars for good stabilization practice.

Elliptical Trainer — A machine with pedals that move in an elliptical cycle and, along with an adjustable incline, simulate running without impact. Some models come with arm levers that alternate, and these are preferable for a good full-body warm-up.

Treadmill — A machine with a moving ramp that can be adjusted to different speeds and inclines for walking and running. Use without holding handrails for good stabilization practice.

Additional beneficial exercise machines for swimmers include:

Swim Bench — Replicates swimming motion, including accelerating movement, and encourages correct technique against more resistance than the water provides. It also encourages the swimmer to accelerate movements throughout each exertion.

Erg — Also known as the rowing machine, the erg builds force and power very well, closely replicating the full-body requirements of rowing, which in many ways are similar to swimming.

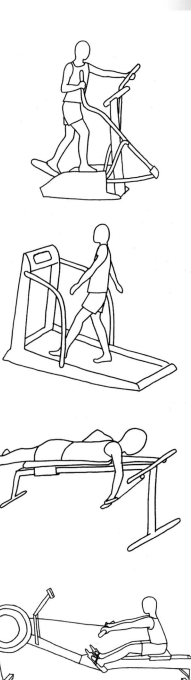

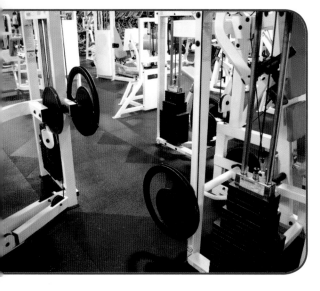

WEIGHTS

Weightlifting is recommended only for athletes who have reached the young adult stage of development. Real consequences can occur when weights are used too early in a swimmer's development. It is not a myth! Growth plates in young developing swimmers can be damaged under the load of weights.

When a swimmer is physically ready for weights, they provide an efficient way to build muscle strength. Weight rooms are full of equipment and machines, some which address swimming and some that don't. It is important to remember that we are trying to simulate swimming movement, directionality and tempo as much as possible.

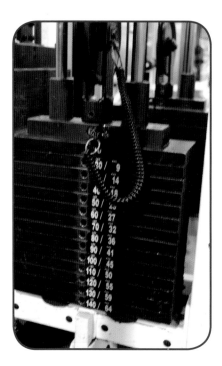

WEIGHT MACHINES

Weight machines that use pulley systems generally address swimming movement in terms of directionality, range of motion, and by requiring accelerating movements. There are also machines that work on lever systems. Some of these are beneficial to swimmers. Some, however, apply resistance in the reverse direction of swimming, and others are designed to isolate muscles rather than to engage multi-muscle movements.

Weight machines that are especially beneficial to swimmers include:

UPPER BODY/ARMS

Lat Pull — This machine has a wide bar suspended overhead from a cable and a pulley that attaches to an adjustable stack of weights at the other end below. To perform this exercise, stand or sit on a bench just inside the bar and grasp it at a point wider than the shoulders. Pull the long handle down 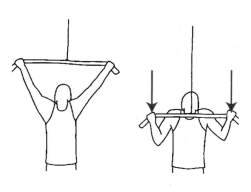 behind the head and recover along the same path. Repeat.
Variation: Stand or sit on a bench just outside the bar and pull the bar down in front to the chest.

Cable Pull — This machine has a bar attached to cables and pulleys that attach to an adjustable stack of weights. Many exercises can be performed on this machine, but two simulate swimming best. The first is done by standing facing the machine, holding the bar with the arms extended overhead, then doing a double arm freestyle underwater pull. The second is done lying on the back on a bench in front of the machine, holding the bar with the arms extended overhead, then a double arm freestyle underwater pull. In both cases, recover along the same path and repeat.

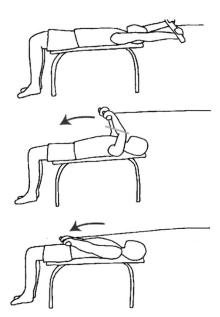

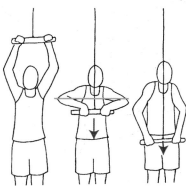

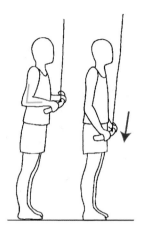

Triceps Press — This machine has a narrow bar suspended overhead from a cable and a pulley that attaches to an adjustable stack of weights at the other end below. To perform this exercise, stand facing the machine and grasp the handle with both hands, holding the elbows at a right angle and firmly at the sides of the body. Press the handle downward and recover along the same path, maintaining firm elbows and wrists. Repeat.

LEGS

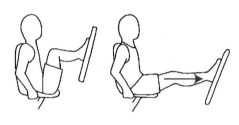

Leg Press — This machine has a seat and a platform for the feet attached to a lever with weights at the other end. To perform this exercise, sit and place the feet on the platform with the seat adjusted so that legs are bent at a 90-degree angle at the knees. Press until the legs are straight. Recover along the same path. Avoid locking the knees. Repeat.

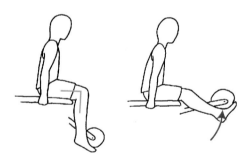

Quad Lift — This machine has a bench attached to a lever with weights on the other end. To perform this exercise, sit on the bench and place the tops of the feet under the lever. Lift until the legs are straight. Recover along the same path. Avoid locking the knees. Repeat.

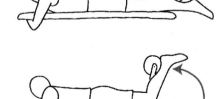

Hamstring Lift — This machine has a bench attached to a lever with weights on the other end. To perform this exercise, lay face down on the bench and place the backs of the ankles under the lever. Raise the feet until the knees are at a right angle. Recover along the same path. Repeat.

FREE WEIGHTS

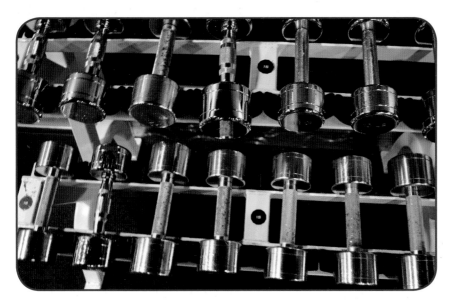

Beyond weight machines, there is also equipment known as free weights. These include hand-held dumbbells, barbells and bars. Work with free weights can be useful as it requires the swimmer to stabilize the weight while exerting. However, many free weight exercises do not address swimming motion as the resistance applied is in the reverse direction of swimming. Free weight activities for swimmers should be carefully evaluated in terms of objective and be included as a primary activity only if they simulate swimming motion.

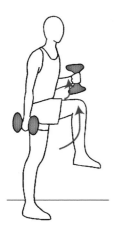

Free weight activities that are especially beneficial to swimmers include:

FULL BODY

March — Stand holding a dumbbell in each hand at your sides. In a thumbs-up position, raise the dumbbell in the left hand to the shoulder. At the same time, raise the knee of the right leg to 90 degrees. Recover along the same path, as the opposite limbs perform the motion. Repeat in a rhythmic, alternating manner.

Squat Jumps — Stand holding a dumbbell in each hand at your sides. Squat, then stand and jump explosively. Repeat.

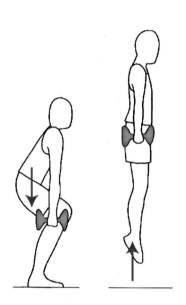

CORE

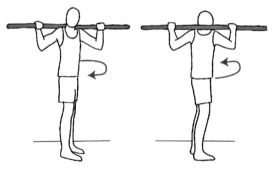

Bar Twists — Standing with feet positioned at least as wide as your shoulders. Hold a long bar behind the shoulders, turn and twist to the right, then to the left repeatedly.

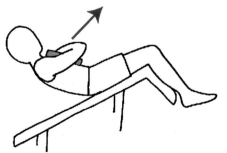

Incline Crunches — Lying face up on an inclined bench, with the head at the lowest point, hold a barbell over the chest and raise your upper body off the bench. Recover along the same path. Repeat.

UPPER BODY/ARMS

Triceps Extension — Using a bench to support your left arm and your left knee, bend forward at the waist. Hold a dumbbell in your right hand, with your arm perpendicular to the surface of the bench. With the palm back, press back like the finish of the freestyle, holding the elbow still. Recover along the same path. Repeat. Do the same exercise with the other arm.

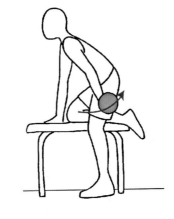

Barbell Curls — Stand with a barbell held with both hands shoulder length apart, palms forward. Raise the barbell to the shoulders without moving the elbows. Recover along the same path. Repeat.

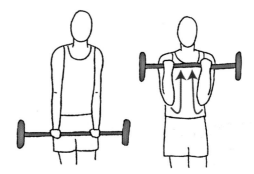

LEGS

Dumbbell Squats — Stand with the feet positioned at least as wide as shoulders. Hold a dumbbell at the sides, looking forward the whole time, and squat until the knees are at a maximum of 90 degrees, then stand. Repeat.

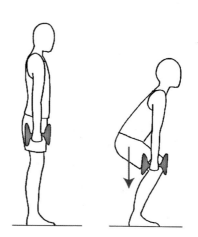

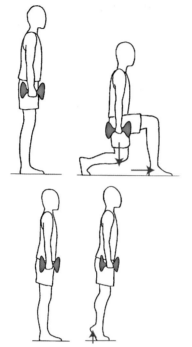

Dumbbell Lunges — Holding a dumbbell in each hand, take a large stride forward, until the trailing knee nearly touches the ground, then stand and bring the trailing leg forward. Repeat, alternating leading legs.

Dumbbell Heel Raises — Stand holding a dumbbell at your sides. Raise both heels off the ground and then lower them. Repeat.

BALANCE

All of the above exercises.

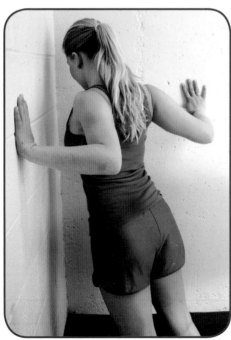

SHOULDER STABILIZATION

These two exercises are to be done with a very small amount of weight. There is no room for "macho" behavior here! Use a weight that is between 1 to 5 pounds only. These exercises are part of a shoulder maintenance routine found on page 157.

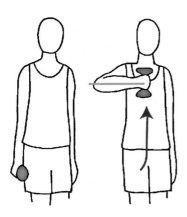

Raise a Glass — Hold a small dumbbell in your left hand, and align your hand with your belly button. With your thumb up, raise your hand and elbow simultaneously as if raising a glass to your mouth. Recover along the same path. Repeat. Perform the same exercise with the other arm.

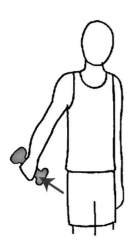

Diagonal Lift — Holding a small dumbbell in your left hand, in the thumbs down position, raise your hand approximately 12 inches along a path that is 45 degrees to the front of the body. Recover along the same path. Repeat. Perform the same exercise with the right arm.

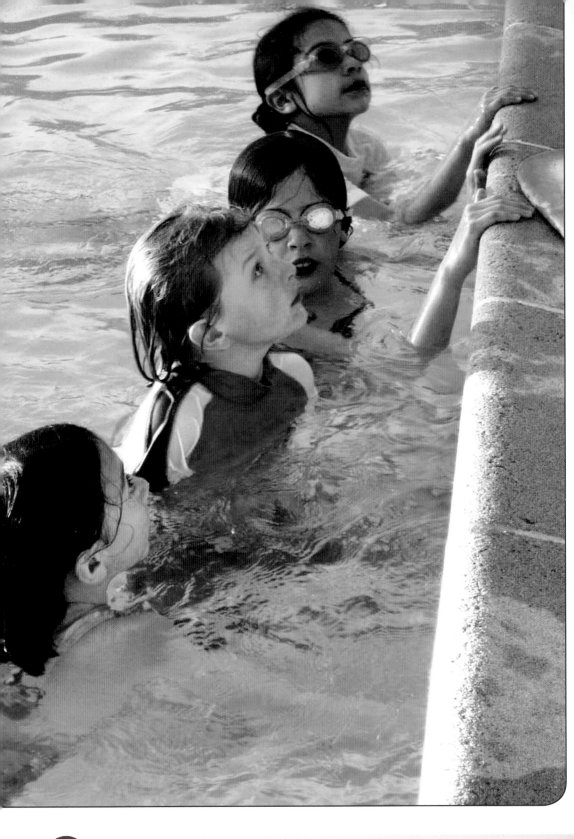

6 THE FUNDAMENTALS

Just as in swimming where you must know how to float right before you can swim right, likewise with strength training, you must have a clear understanding of the basics before you can gain the results of faster swimming. Fundamental principles represent the foundation from which you can structure a program that will have predictable and positive results.

HOW MUCH AND HOW MANY?

These are very important questions when it comes to strength training. We must clearly understand the significance of how much resistance, how many repetitions, at what rate, and how much frequency and duration is necessary in relation to our strength training objectives. Without this knowledge, we could end up with a different outcome than intended. More quantity does not always translate to more strength. Knowing "how much" and "how many" is as important as knowing which exercises to do.

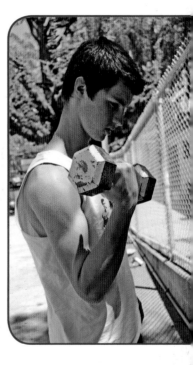

HOW MUCH RESISTANCE?

With self-resistance work, the load that is resisted is exclusively the swimmer's body weight, but when external load is added, as with stretch cords, medicine balls and weights, the question of how much resistance needs to be answered. In general, to build power, the athlete should be able to repeat the exercise with a load 12 to 15 times without failure. If he or she cannot do this, the load is too much. If it is extremely easy, the load is too little. In contrast, to build force, a larger load should be used. The athlete should be able to repeat an exercise only about three to five times. Again, if he or she cannot do this, the load is too much. If it is extremely easy, the load is too little.

HOW MANY REPETITIONS?

We also need to know how many times to repeat a particular action or sequence. We count repetitions, or reps, and we count sets. A rep is a single action of the exercise. Use the guidelines described above for reps. A set is a group of reps. Multiple sets have rest between them. As far as how many sets to do, when the objective is force or explosiveness, fewer sets are done, and sometimes, only a single set is performed. When the objective is power or endurance, more sets are done. Most people do three to five sets when training for power.

HOW MUCH RATE?

How fast or slowly an exercise is repeated also is determined by the strength training objective. An exercise done at a faster rate tends to build force and explosiveness. An exercise done at slower rate tends to build power.

With some exercises, it is possible to simulate swimming tempo very well by allowing the athlete to perform repetitions at a rate of about one per second. Stretch cord work is a good example of this. Some exercises are not designed for stroke tempo work, so do not attempt to achieve such a tempo. The Lat Pull is a good example of an exercise that should not be used for tempo work as it is very important not to rush the recovery, but to control it instead.

HOW RESISTANCE, REPETITIONS AND RATE WORK TOGETHER

To get the intended outcome, we look at the amount of resistance, or load, the number of repetitions and sets, and the rate that the exercise is performed together. For instance, if our objective is to develop force, we must pair fewer repetitions and sets with more load. If we try to build force by increasing both the number of repetitions and the load at the same time, the swimmer will soon experience failure, and the objective will not be met. In contrast, if our objective is to develop power, we must pair more repetitions and sets with less resistance. If we try to build power by increasing both the number of repetitions and the load at the same time, the swimmer will soon experience failure, and the objective will not be met.

HOW MUCH FREQUENCY AND DURATION?

Frequency refers to the number of strength training sessions in a week, month or season. Duration refers to how long each session is. Frequency should be determined by the swimmer's stage of development in conjunction with the strength training content. For instance, a program using weights, for developmentally advanced swimmers should accommodate rest and recovery time between sessions. A program for beginners, however, that is based on a good variety of self-resistance activities can be done several days in a row in order to develop a good athletic base. Swimmers in the adult or senior stages of development should build in more rest days, as recovery takes longer.

BEFORE OR AFTER SWIMMING?

When is the best time to do strength training, before or after swimming? The debate is ongoing.

On the one hand, it is clear that strength training before swimming activates the muscles that will be used in the pool. Swimming-specific strength training before swimming also reinforces good form in the water. Studies have shown that the nervous system connections established and practiced on land carry over to stroke actions in the pool when swimming directly follows land activities. Finally, many believe that swimmers who swim regularly after a strength training develop better endurance, as swimming, which builds endurance very well, becomes an extension of a "super workout" begun on land, requiring the swimmer to adapt to a greater workload.

On the other hand, some believe that since swimming elongates the muscles, strength work that follows swimming ensures that the swimmer's muscles are well warmed up and less vulnerable to injury from the demands of land training. They also argue that when strength training follows the water workout, the quality of the swimming is higher because a swimmer who is tired after strength training practices swimming slower, with less force, power and explosiveness, reinforcing undesirable habits. Finally, many take the position that swimming first allows the swimmer to feel and utilize the strength that he or she has adapted to in the water where it counts.

So which is best? There are valid arguments for both. From the perspective of preparing a swimmer to race, to be ready to perform under less than ideal conditions, including poor weather, crowded warm-up areas and meet delays, a program that uses a bit of both approaches should be considered. By mixing it up, the swimmer will practice adapting to different situations. Further, changing the order of the training routine from time to time will keep it from becoming boring, as the swimmer will stay challenged to perform under different circumstances.

The final decision should be based on what best works for the individual athlete.

Scheduling rest time is as important as scheduling workout time. Even routines based solely on self-resistance work should allow at least two days off per week. When the content of the strength work includes external load, at least three rest days are recommended. A routine of alternating work days and rest days works well. Some athletes use a daily schedule, by alternating days for upper body and lower body. Attention should be paid to levels of fatigue when using this model. A schedule of two work days in a row, followed by one rest day has also proven successful. The particular schedule should consider the rest requirements of the individual swimmer, assuming he or she is swimming five to six days a week.

The duration of each strength training session should also be determined by a swimmer's particular stage of development, as well as his or her swimming experience. In the early stages, sessions should be quite short because not a great deal of endurance has been developed. Still, a lot of work can be accomplished in 15 to 30 minutes! As the swimmer matures physically, longer training sessions of an hour or more are beneficial, both because the swimmer is capable of more and because more types of activities, more repetitions, and more sets take more time.

Answering these fundamental questions must be done before strength training begins. To achieve more swimming speed, careful analysis of "how much and how many" should be done with the specific objective of the swimmer in mind.

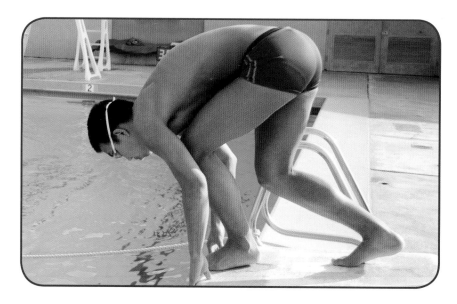

START RIGHT

SAFETY

Like the "No Diving" sign at the shallow end of the pool, safety rules are there for a reason. Although you may be lucky diving into shallow water, the consequences are real and grave. When safety rules for conduct and equipment use are in place, observe them with respect. If safety rules are not in place, it is the responsibility of the supervisor to establish them.

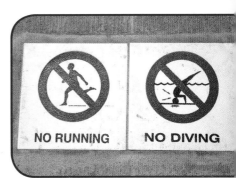

Supervision is a must, especially when children and inexperienced swimmers are engaged in strength training activities. The supervisor must ensure that safety rules are understood and followed. The supervisor must ensure that each activity is performed correctly and safely by each swimmer. The supervisor must ensure that each activity is appropriate for the swimmer's stage of development and experience.

Everyone engaged in strength training should use a proactive approach to preventing accidents by:

Training With a Partner

All strength training, especially with weights, should be done with a partner who can spot and assist, and observe technique.

Handling Weights Correctly

Lift weights from the floor using your legs rather than your back. Weights should never be dropped; hey can break bones. They should also not be left on the floor to trip on. Medicine balls should never be thrown at the face or the groin, only at the chest and when the person is looking.

Wearing Shoes

Although most swimmers are very comfortable in bare feet around the pool deck, shoes should be mandatory for any strength training activity involving external weight or moving with impact on the feet. While many exercises can be done safely without shoes on the pool deck or gym, it is never acceptable to be barefoot in the weight room where obstacles are many or when using any exercise machine with moving parts. Self-resistance work that involves running, jumping, or changing directions can put excessive pressure on bare feet. Shoes will provide support as well as protection from sharp objects hidden in grass and rough surfaces.

Tying Hair Back

Long hair back should be tied back to ensure good visibility at all times and to avoid entanglement in machines.

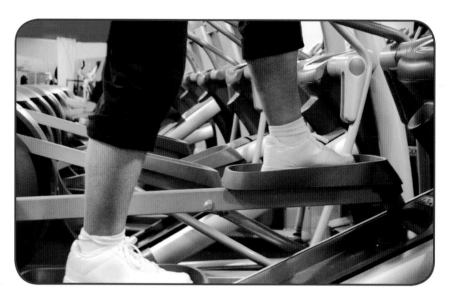

WARM-UP

The purpose of warming up before strength training is exactly the same as at the beginning of a swimming workout. Warming up prepares the body to work by loosening up and activating the muscles, and raising the heart rate to circulate oxygen-rich blood to the muscles. Swimmers should spend at least a quarter of their strength training time warming up.

Good warm-up activities include:
- Relaxed Arm Circles
- Hanging Arm Circles
- Cherry Pickers
- Jumping Jacks
- Running
- Skipping
- Side Steps
- Stairs
- Skating
- Jump Rope

TAKE IT EASY ON THE STRETCHING!

Stretching has long been a traditional part of warming up before exercise, but the fact is, stretching has injured many swimmers. There are two reasons for this:

1. Stretching does not prepare the body to work, as a warm-up should do. By using valuable warm-up time for stretching, a swimmer runs out of time to do activities that raise the heart rate and activate the muscles. Beginning a workout in this state leaves the body more prone to injury. In addition, without a good warm-up, some or all of the workout is wasted because the swimmer is not prepared to exert.

2. In general, swimmers have very mobile joints, so stretching is really unnecessary. This is especially true of shoulder stretching. Because the shoulders are so central to swimming, they are commonly the site of soreness for many swimmers. In an effort to relieve soreness, we turn to stretching. But what happens when these muscles are stretched is that too much looseness develops, which can lead to joint stability problems during swimming, producing more soreness and pain.

Instead of stretching as a warm-up, swimmers should spend warm-up time doing full-body activity with gradually progressive effort. As far as the shoulders, rather than stretching, the focus should be on stabilizing mobility at the joints to keep them operating correctly. This is done through specific shoulder stabilization exercises, as shown on page 94-95.

If stretching is done at all, it should be done after exercise. It should be very conservative and target only the large muscles, not the joints. Even this kind of stretching should be gentle and gradual. Under no circumstances should any bouncing action be used. Under no circumstances should another swimmer apply external stretching pressure for you. Under no circumstances should stretching hurt, either during or after you do it.

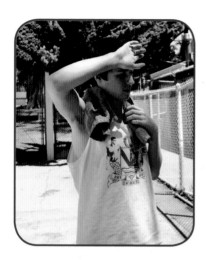

When exercise machines are available, warm-ups can include:
- Exercise Bike
- Elliptical Trainer
- Treadmill

COOL DOWN

Just as after swimming, the cool down is important to let body systems and muscles adjust to the resting state. After exercise, allow several minutes of slow, continuous activity so the heart rate can return to normal and the muscles can begin to relax. One of the best cool down activities is walking.

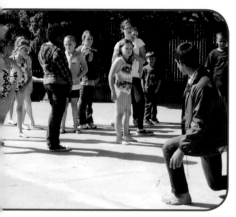

FORM

Form is as important in strength training as it is in the water. Form determines the manner in which the swimmer's body interacts with the resistance. It is important to spend time perfecting the swimmer's form on any particular exercise before it is repeated over and over. Correct form ensures that the swimmer will use the intended muscles groups in the intended fashion. Incorrect form can lead to poor results, including injury.

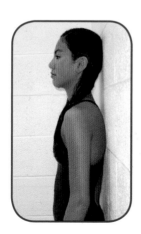

POSTURE

Our symmetrical bodies are designed with many bilateral muscles, including the lats, the obliques, the pectoralis major and the deltoids, among others. However, when one part of our body is out of alignment, the mirror image muscles are very adept at taking over the work. Repeated exercise with poor posture can result in bilateral muscles developing unevenly as one side compensates for the other. As swimming depends on bilateral strength, maintaining good posture is very important.

Good posture starts with the awareness of your body position and stance. One of the most positive steps you can take is to develop core strength that stabilizes posture from the front and the back. This will help keep shoulders, hips and knees in alignment, encouraging strength to be developed in a more balanced manner.

BREATHING

Breathing function is an essential part of athletic performance. Posture plays an important part in good breathing function. Bad posture encumbers breathing capacity by allowing the trunk of the body to be compressed, leaving less room for the lungs to expand and contract. One of the quickest and best ways to improve your breathing during exercise is to stand up straight.

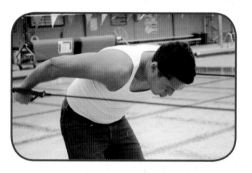

Breathing rhythm is very important. Just as we use rhythmic breathing in the pool, it should also be used during strength training. Avoid holding the breath during exertion. Instead, just like swimming, and most all other sports, exhale during exertion and inhale during recovery. Exchanging air properly will keep your muscles better supplied with the oxygen they need to perform. It will also keep you from fatiguing as quickly.

CONTROL

It is important to control every movement against resistance, both in the power phase and recovery. Always maintain balance and stability during the power phase. Always return to the starting position gently and with less speed. Never allow an external load to jerk the limbs back to the starting position.

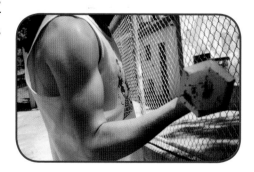

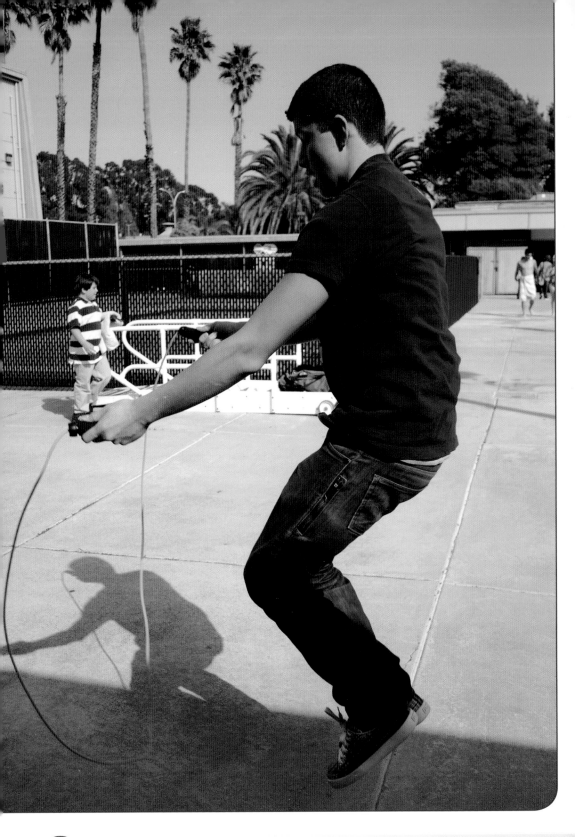

7 ROUTINES AND CIRCUITS

This section contains strength training routines and circuits for all stages of development. Because the six stages of development identified earlier in this book are not isolated but are more of a continuum, merging one into the next, the routines and circuits are presented in four progressive levels with specific content to meet particular developmental objectives. Use these routines and circuits as examples for structure and content, then tailor them to the needs of the individual swimmer.

Check with your health care provider before starting a strength training program.

STRENGTH TRAINING ROUTINES

The following routines are presented in a sequence beginning with a warm-up and ending with a cool down. When a double space appears, extra rest should be taken.

LEVEL 1	LEVEL 2	LEVEL 3	LEVEL 4
ELEMENTARY			
PRE-ADOLESCENCE			
	ADOLESCENCE		
		YOUNG ADULT	
		ADULT	
	SENIOR		

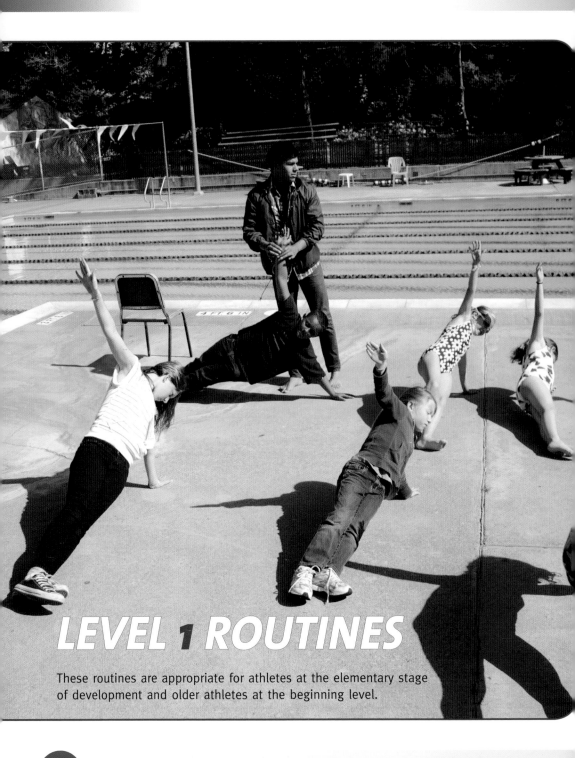

LEVEL 1 ROUTINES

These routines are appropriate for athletes at the elementary stage of development and older athletes at the beginning level.

1Routine

Approximately 15 minutes
Objective: General athleticism

Warm-up:
10 Arm Circles (front)
10 Arm Circles (back)
10 Cherry Pickers
25 Jumping Jacks

25 Crunches
30 Seconds of Air Kicking
30 Seconds of Plank

50 Streamlined Leaps
30 Lunges
10 Shoulder Shrugs

Skipping Relays
Crawling Relays

Cool down:
2 minutes of Walking

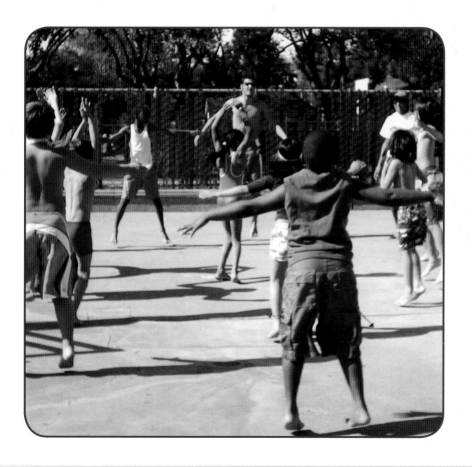

2Routine

Approximately 15 minutes
Objective: General athleticism

Warm-up:
2 minutes of Skipping
3 minutes of Hula Hoop

10 Burpies
25 Chest Lifts
10 Burpies
25 Left, Right, Ups
10 Burpies

1 minute of Streamlined Leaps
3 minutes of Net Climbing

Cool down:
2 minutes of Walking

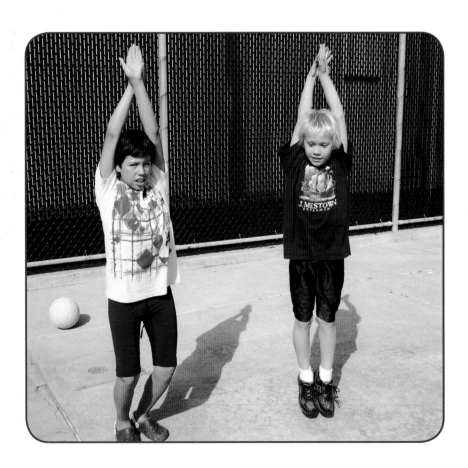

3Routine

Approximately 15 minutes
Objective: General athleticism

Warm-up:
100 Quick Jump Ropes

30 seconds of Insect
1 minute of Crab Walking
30 seconds of Plank

1 minute of Side Steps
1 minute of Balance Ball Crunches

2 minutes of Cartwheels
2 minutes of Running Stairs

Cool down:
2 minutes of Walking

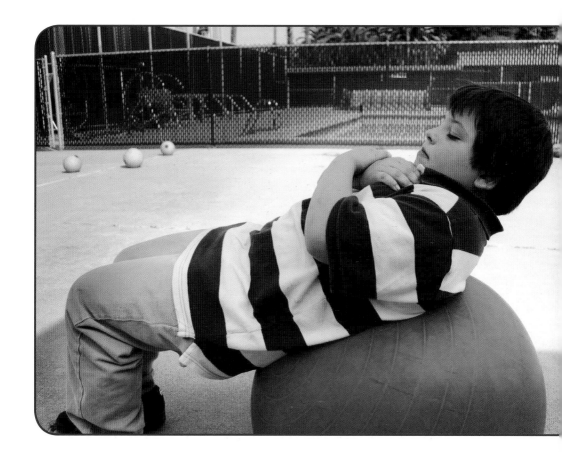

4 Routine

Approximately 15 minutes
Objective: General athleticism

Warm-up:
25 Jumping Jacks
30 seconds of One Leg Balancing
25 Jumping Jacks
30 seconds of Alternating Extensions
25 Jumping Jacks

10 Bleacher Dips
20 Streamlined Leaps
30 Shrugs
40 Lunges

3 minutes of Zig Zags

Cool down:
2 minutes of Walking

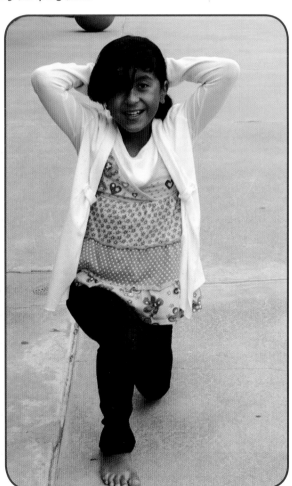

5Routine

Approximately 15 minutes
Objective: General athleticism

Warm-up:
10 Arm Circles (front)
10 Arm Circles (back)
10 Shrugs
3 minutes of Running Lines

3 minutes of Net Climbing

20 Balance Ball Chest Lifts
30 seconds of High Plank
10 Box Jumps
2 minutes Speed Jump roping

Cool down:
2 minutes of Walking

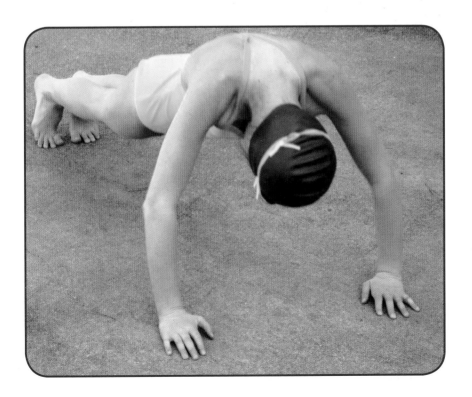

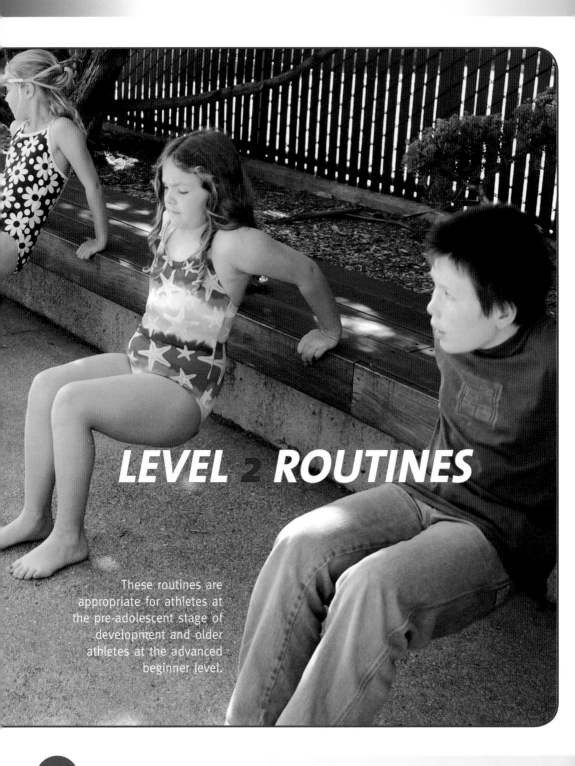

LEVEL 2 ROUTINES

These routines are appropriate for athletes at the pre-adolescent stage of development and older athletes at the advanced beginner level.

6 Routine

Approximately 20 minutes
Objective: Power/Stability

Warm-up:
3 minutes of Jump Rope
50 Jumping Jacks
10 Cherry Pickers

25 Balance Ball Crunches
25 Balance Ball Chest Lifts
10 Bleacher Dips
1 minute of Streamline Leaps

30 seconds of Plank
30 seconds of Side Plank (left)

30 seconds of Side Plank (right)

20 Alternating Extensions
1 minute of Air Kicking
1 minute of Body Lifts

30 Box Jumps
1 minute of One Leg Balancing

Cool down:
2 minutes of Walking

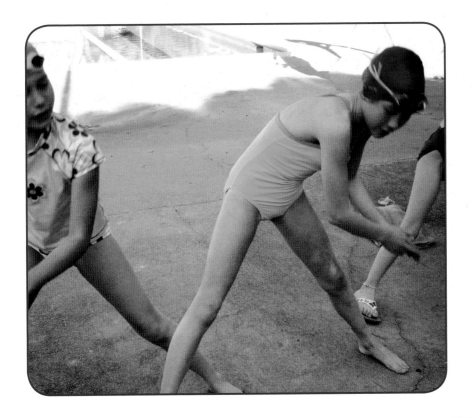

7 Routine

**Approximately 20 minutes
Objective: Power/Coordination**

Warm-up:
2 minutes of Running Lines
1 minute of Skipping
1 minute of Side Steps
1 minute of Cherry Pickers

3 minutes of Rope Climbing
20 Bleacher Dips
20 Corner Push-ups
3 minutes of Net Climbing

25 V Ups
1 minute of Air Kicking
25 Leg Crosses
1 minute of Balance Ball Passes

1 minute of Quick Clap

Cool down:
2 minutes of walking

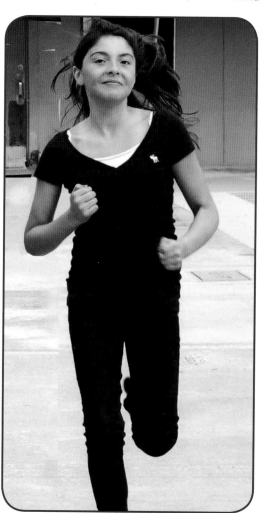

8 Routine

**Approximately 20 minutes
Objective: Coordination/Tempo**

Warm-up:
50 Jumping Jacks
2 minutes of Stairs
1 minute of Speed Walking

30 Balance Ball Crunches
30 Balance Ball Chest Lifts
1 minute of Alternating
Limb Balance

20 Shrugs
20 Arm Circles (front)
20 Arm Circles (back)

10 Body Lifts
20 Streamlined Leaps
30 Bleacher Dips
40 Lunges

1 minute of Skipping
1 minute of Crab Walk
1 minute of Crawling
2 minutes of Speed Jump Rope

Cool down:
2 minutes of Walking

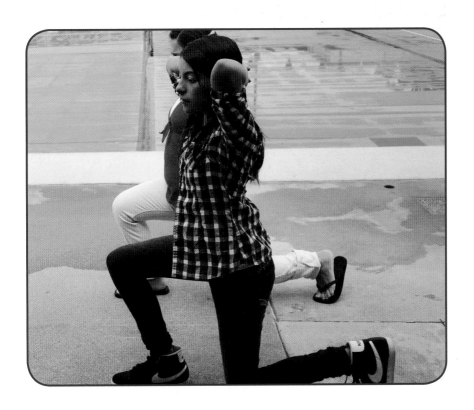

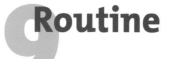Routine

Approximately 20 minutes
Objective: Power

Warm-up:
20 Burpies
1 minute of Skipping
1 minute of Speed Walking
20 Burpies

1 minute of Plank
30 seconds of High Side Plank (left)
30 seconds of High Side Plank (right)

1 minute of Leg Crosses

1 minute of Stairs

1 minute of Leg Crosses
30 Bleacher Dips
30 Box Jumps

3 minutes of Net Climbing

Cool down:
2 minutes of Walking

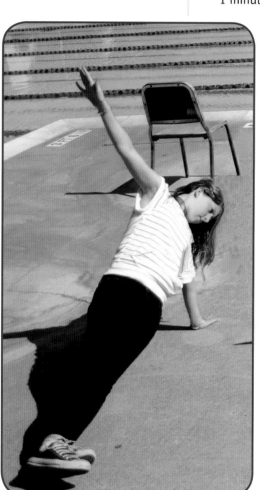

10 Routine

Approximately 20 minutes
Objective: Power/Stability

Warm-up:
5 minutes of Running
1 minute of Quick Clap

With Balance Ball:
30 Ball Crunches
30 Chest Lifts
30 seconds Streamline
1 minute of Balance Ball Passes
30 seconds Single Leg Balance
(front – right)

30 seconds Single Leg Balance
(front – left)

25 Jumping Jacks
25 Streamlined Leaps
25 Lunges
25 Burpies

3 minutes of Rope Climbing

Cool down:
2 minutes of Walking

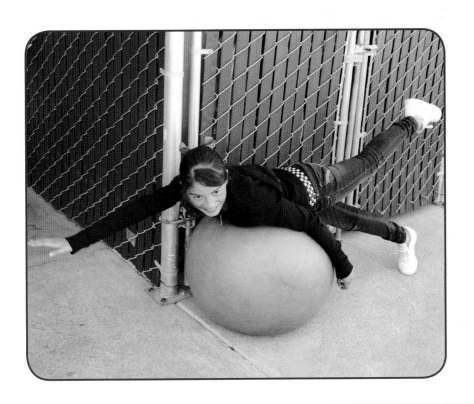

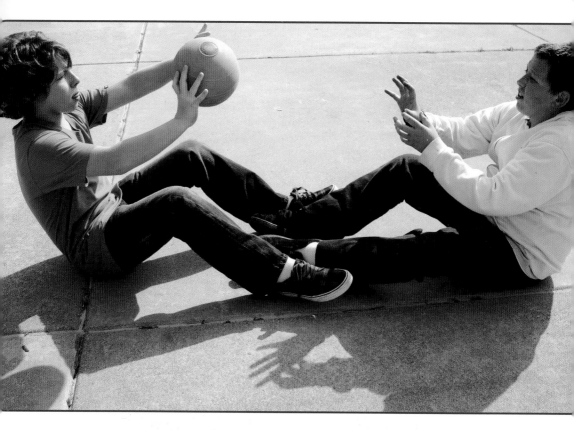

LEVEL 3 ROUTINES

These routines are appropriate for athletes at the adolescent stage of development and older athletes at the intermediate level.

11 Routine

Approximately 30 minutes
Objective: Power/Stability

Warm-up:
3 minutes of Jump Rope
2 minutes of Stairs
2 minutes of Speed Jump Rope
3 minutes of Stairs

3 Sets with Medicine Ball:
30 Left, Right, Ups
1 minute of Standing Rebounds
30 Squats

3 Sets with Stretch Cord - increasing tempo each set:
1 minute of Double Arm Pull
1 minute of Triceps Press

1 minute of Insect
1 minute of Plank
30 seconds of Side Plank (left)
30 seconds of Side Plank (right)

Cool down:
3 minutes of Walking

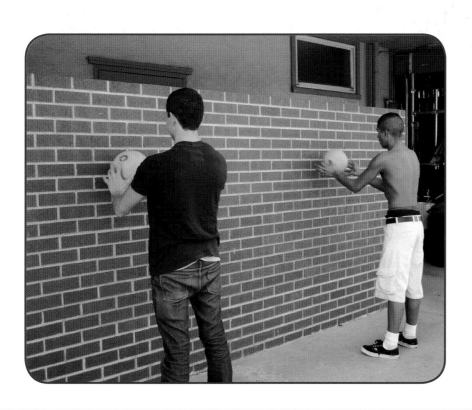

12 Routine

Approximately 30 minutes
Objective: Power/Tempo

Warm-up:
25 Burpies
5 minutes of Running

1 minute of Hand Switch
1 minute of Quick Clap
30 Bleacher Dips
30 Corner Push Outs

50 Streamline Leaps

2 Sets with Medicine Ball:
1 minute of Squats
3 minutes of Quick Toss
with Partner

1 minute of Squats
1 minute of Hike with Partner

2 Sets with Balance Ball:
50 Crunches
50 Chest Lifts
1 minute of Alternating
Limb Balance

2 minutes of Stairs

Cool down:
3 minutes of Walking

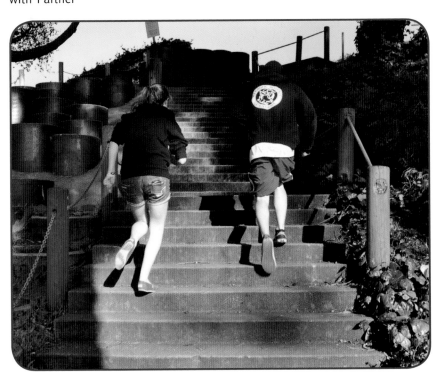

13 Routine

Approximately 30 minutes
Objective: Force/Stability

Warm-up:
3 minutes of Running Lines
1 minute of Hand Switch
2 minutes of Speed Walking
1 minute of Quick Clap
3 minutes of Running Lines

3 Sets with Stretch Band:
1 minute of Double Arm Pull
1 minute of Alternating
Arm Pull
1 minute of Double
Triceps Press

1 minute Plank
1 minute of Leg Crosses
30 V Ups

3 Sets with Medicine Ball:
30 Left, Right, Ups
30 Standing Wall Rebounds
30 Leg Lift and Pass

3 minutes of Stairs

Cool down:
3 minutes of Walking

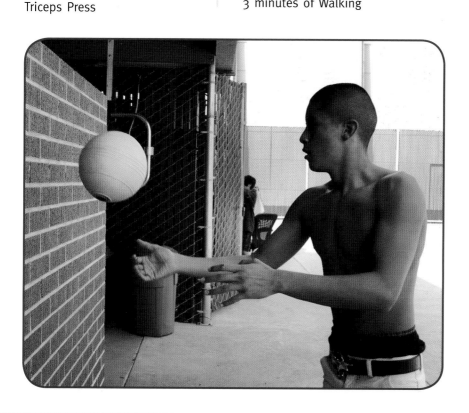

14 Routine

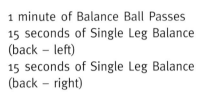

**Approximately 30 minutes
Objective: Force/Stability**

Warm-up:
4 minutes of Lines
3 minutes of Skipping
2 minutes of Zig Zags
1 minute of Streamlined Leaps
30 seconds of Frog Jumps

With Balance Ball:
50 Crunches
50 Chest Lifts
15 seconds of Single Leg Balance
(front − left)
15 seconds of Single Leg Balance
(front − right)

1 minute of Balance Ball Passes
15 seconds of Single Leg Balance
(back − left)
15 seconds of Single Leg Balance
(back − right)

2 minutes Double Arm Pull with
Stretch Cord
2 minutes of Quick Toss with
Medicine Ball with Partner
2 minutes of Alternating Arm Pull
with Stretch Cord
2 minutes of Quick Toss with
Medicine Ball with Partner

With Balance Ball:
50 Crunches
50 Chest Lifts
15 seconds of Single Leg Balance
(front − left)
15 seconds of Single Leg Balance
(front − right)
1 minute of Balance Ball Passes
15 seconds of Single Leg Balance
(back − left)
15 seconds of Single Leg Balance
(back − right)

3 minutes of Rope Climbing
3 minutes of Net Climbing

Cool down:
3 minutes of Walking

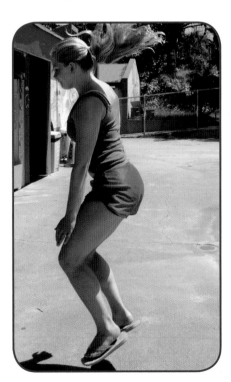

15 **Routine**

Approximately 30 minutes
Objective: Force/Power

Warm-up:
3 minutes of Jump Rope
20 Burpies
10 Arm Circles (left)
10 Arm Circles (right)
1 minute of Streamlined Leaps
3 minutes of Stretch Cord –
Alternating Arms

2 Sets with Medicine Ball:
2 minutes of Pass Around
with Partner

2 minutes of Quick Toss
with Partner
2 minutes of Crunch Toss
with Partner

50 Lunges
1 minute of Leg Crosses
50 Lunges
1 minute of Plank

Cool down:
3 minutes of Walking

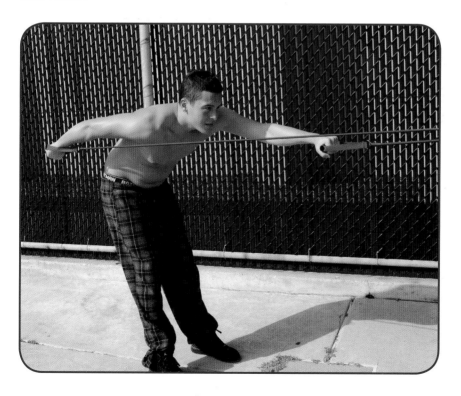

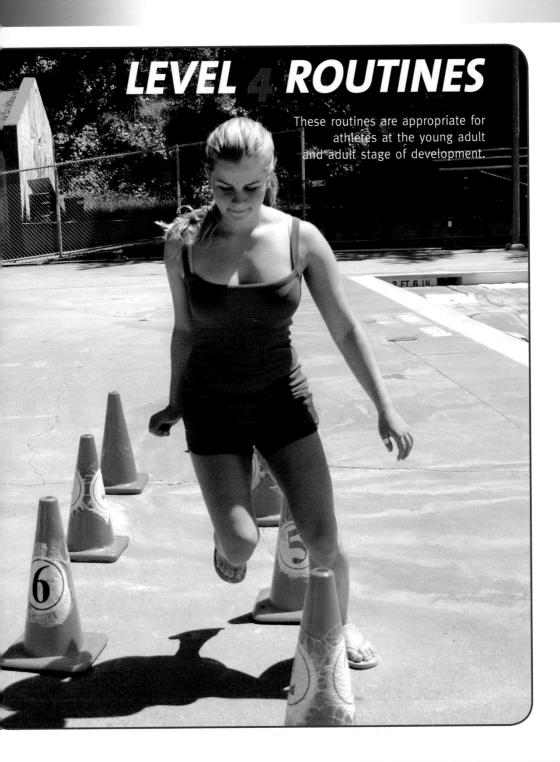

LEVEL 4 ROUTINES

These routines are appropriate for athletes at the young adult and adult stage of development.

16 Routine

Approximately 1 hour
Objective: Power/Force

Warm-up:
15 minutes on Elliptical Trainer
5 minutes Quick Toss with Partner
1 minute of Box Jumps

3 sets of 12:
Bar Squats
March

3 sets of 12:
Lat Pull
Triceps Press

3 sets of 12:
Leg Press
Toe Raises

1 set of 12:
Dumbbell Curls

1 minute of Plank
30 seconds of High Side Plank (left)
30 seconds of High Side Plank (right)
50 Sky Crunches
1 minute of Air Kicking
1 minute of Balance Ball Passes
3 minutes on Erg

Cool down:
5 minutes of Walking

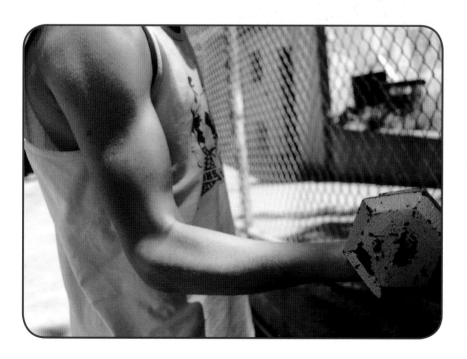

17 Routine

Approximately 1 hour
Objective: Power/Force

Warm-up:
15 minutes on Exercise Bike

With Medicine Ball:
3 minutes of Wall Rebounds (standing)
30 Squat and Jumps
30 Pass Arounds with Partner
2 minutes of Crunch Toss with Partner

With Stretch Cord:
3 minutes of Double Arm Pull
3 minutes of Alternating Arm Pull

2 minutes of Double Arm Pull
2 minutes of Alternating Arm Pull
1 minute of Double Arm Pull
1 minute of Alternating Arm Pull

30 seconds of Peg Board

3 sets of 6:
Quad Lift
Hamstring Press
Bar Squats

5 Frog Leaps

5 minutes of Running Lines
5 minutes of Rope Climbing

Cool down:
5 minutes of Walking

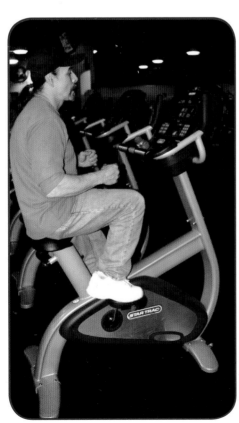

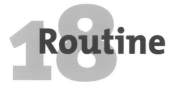

Routine

Approximately 1 hour
Objective: Force/Explosiveness

Warm-up:
15 minutes on Treadmill
2 minutes of Zig Zags
30 Lunges
30 Streamline Leaps

With Medicine Ball:
3 minutes of Quick Toss with Partner
1 minute of Squat and Jump

3 sets of 6:
Lat Pull
Leg Press
Cable Pull

Quad Lift
Triceps Press
Hamstring Lift
2 minutes of Incline Crunches with Weight
1 minute of High Plank
25 Box Jumps
1 minute of Peg Board

1 minute of Quick Clap
5 Frog Jumps

Cool down:
5 minutes of Walking

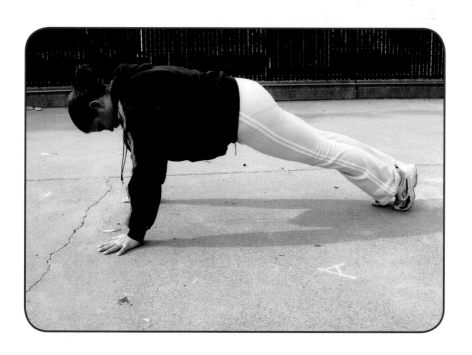

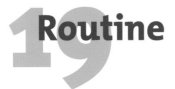

Routine 19

Approximately 1 hour
Objective: Force/Power

Warm-up:
15 minutes on Exercise Bike
15 minutes on Swim Bench

50 Balance Ball Crunches
20 Squats with Medicine Ball
40 Insects
20 Squats with Medicine Ball
30 Left, Right, Ups
20 Squats with Medicine Ball
20 V Ups
20 Squats with Medicine Ball
10 Dumbbell Lunges

1 minute of Speed Jump Rope
3 minutes Rope Climbing
1 minute of Speed Jump Rope

Cool down:
5 minutes of Walking

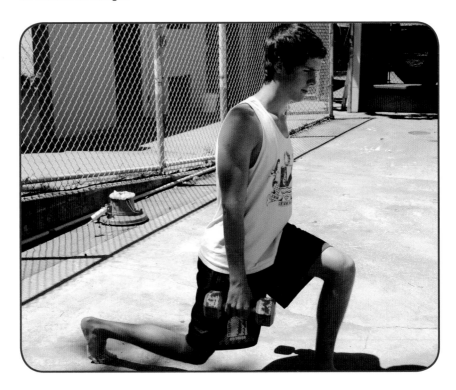

20 Routine

Approximately 1 hour
Objective: Force/Power

Warm-up:
10 minutes of Running
5 minutes of Running Lines

2 minutes of Zig Zags
2 minutes of Skipping
2 minutes of Crab Walk

3 sets of:
6 Lat Pull
6 Triceps Press
3 minutes of Medicine Ball Quick
Toss with Partner

3 sets of:
12 Bar Twists
12 Leg Press
1 minute of Plank

3 sets of:
12 March
12 Burpies
1 minute of Air Kicking

Cool down:
5 minutes of Walking

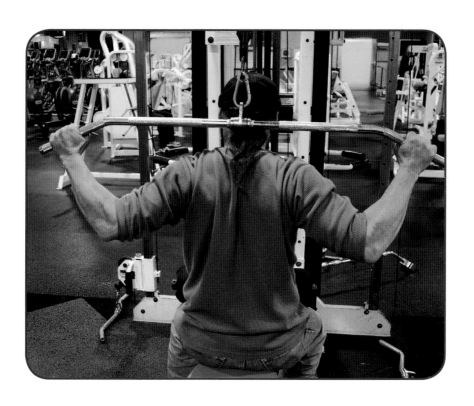

STRENGTH TRAINING CIRCUITS

Circuits are made up of a series of exercise stations that are performed on a time interval. The swimmer goes from one exercise to another without resting. As much work as possible should be performed at a station during the time interval. A swimmer may work through the circuit alone or there can be a swimmer at each station. A good warm-up should be done before beginning the circuit. Circuits are very flexible, as more swimmers can be accommodated easily by adding stations.

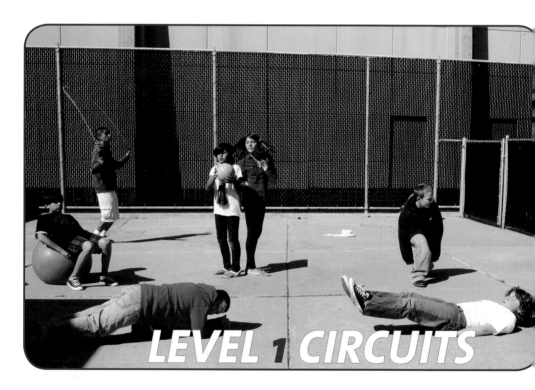

These circuits are appropriate for athletes at the elementary and pre-adolescent stages of development, and older athletes at the beginning level.

1Circuit

Approximately 15 minutes
Objective: General athleticism

Warm-up:
4 minutes of Running

TEN 1-MINUTE STATIONS:
1. Streamlined Leaps
2. Corner Push Outs
3. Insects
4. Box Jumps
5. Bleacher Dips
6. Plank
7. Speed Jump Rope
8. Body Lifts
9. Balance Ball Chest Lifts
10. Burpies

Cool down:
1 minute of Walking

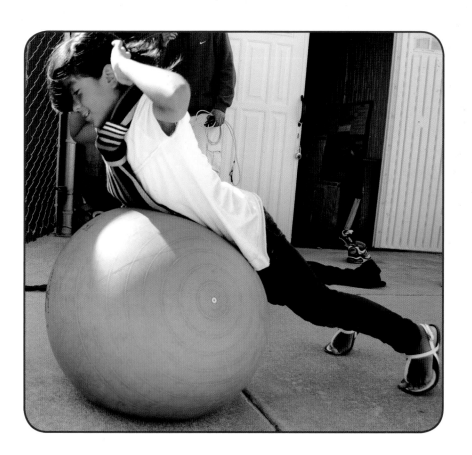

2 Circuit

**Approximately 15 minutes
Objective: General athleticism**

Warm-up:
1 minute of Arm Circles (left and right)
50 Jumping Jacks
1 minute of Quick Clap

TEN 1-MINUTE STATIONS:
1. Hand Switch
2. Streamlined Leaps
3. Air Kicking
4. Corner Push Outs
5. Squats
6. Leg Crosses
7. Burpies
8. Lunges
9. Frog Jumps
10. Plank

Cool down:
1 minute of Walking

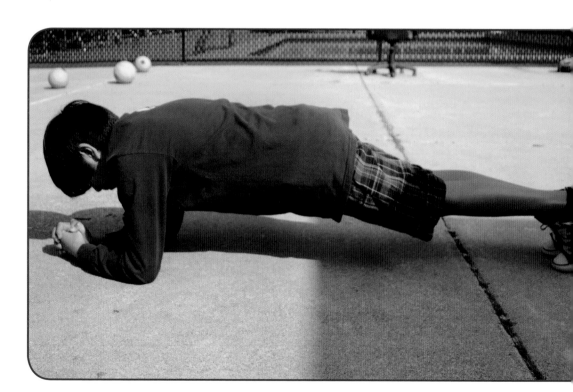

3 Circuit

Approximately 15 minutes
Objective: General athleticism

Warm-up:
2 minutes of Running Lines
1 minute of Cherry Pickers
1 minute of Skipping

TEN 1-MINUTE STATIONS:
1. Jumping Jacks
2. Balance Ball Passes
3. Corner Push Outs
4. Burpies
5. Balance Ball Crunches
6. Lunges
7. Speed Jump Rope
8. V Ups
9. Box Jumps
10. Plank

Cool down:
1 minute of Walking

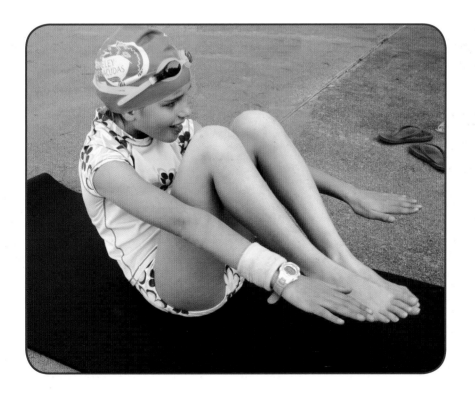

4 Circuit

Approximately 15 minutes
Objective: General athleticism

Warm-up:
1 minute of Arm Circles (left then right)
2 minutes of Running
1 minute of Zig Zags

Cool down:
1 minute of Walking

TEN 1-MINUTE STATIONS:
1. Speed Jump Rope
2. Balance Ball Crunches
3. Corner Push Outs
4. Cherry Pickers
5. Balance Ball Chest Lifts
6. Bleacher Dips
7. Frog Jumps
8. Leg Crosses
9. Plank
10. Lunges

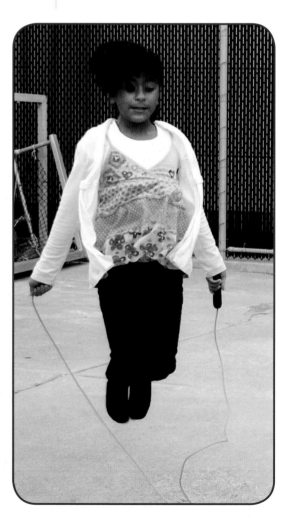

5 Circuit

Approximately 15 minutes
Objective: General athleticism

Warm-up:
3 minutes of Stairs

TEN 1-MINUTE STATIONS:
1. Jumping Jacks
2. Single Leg Balance
3. Balance Ball Crunches
4. Speed Jump Rope
5. Body Lifts
6. Plank
7. Leg Lift and Pass
8. V Ups
9. Balance Ball Alternating Leg Balance
10. Frog Jumps

Cool down:
1 minute of Walking

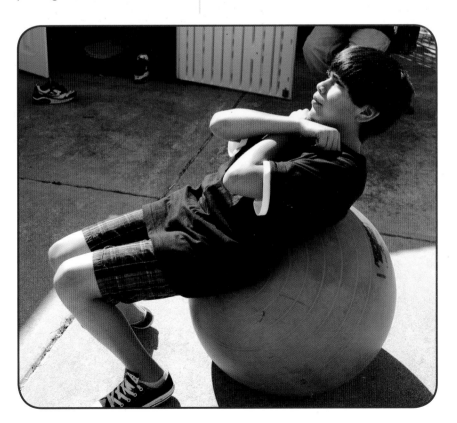

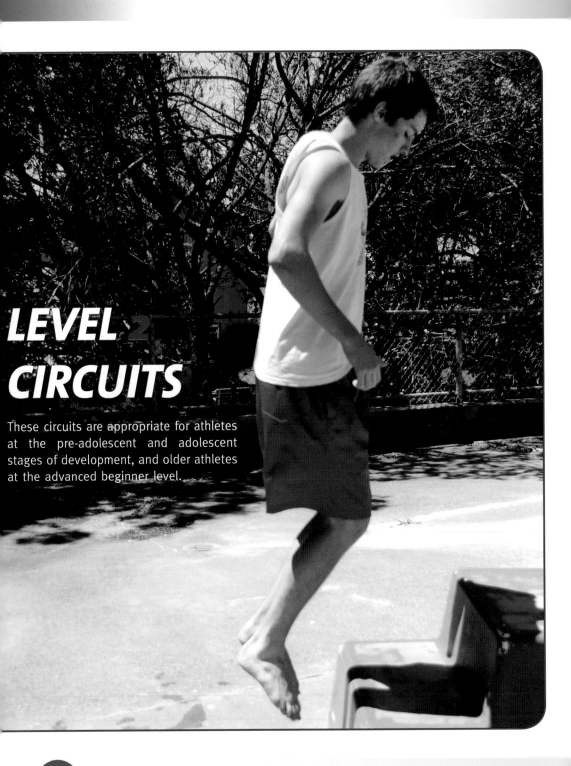

LEVEL 2 CIRCUITS

These circuits are appropriate for athletes at the pre-adolescent and adolescent stages of development, and older athletes at the advanced beginner level.

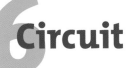

6 Circuit

**Approximately 20 minutes
Objective: Power/Coordination**

Warm-up:
2 minutes of Running
1 minute of Speed Walking

TEN 90-SECOND STATIONS:
1. Streamlined Leaps
2. Bleacher Dips
3. Balance Ball Passes
4. Squats
5. Body Lifts
6. Plank
7. Box Jumps
8. Corner Push Outs
9. Left, Right, Ups
10. Cartwheels

Cool down:
2 minutes of Walking

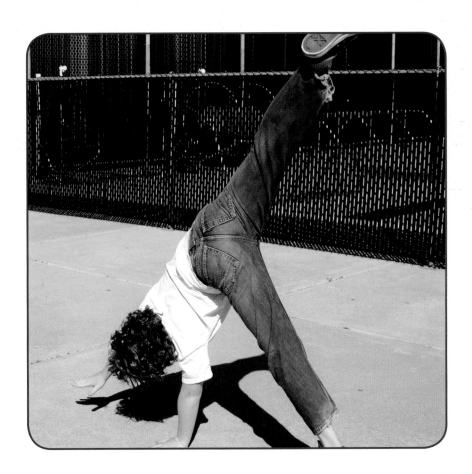

7 Circuit

Approximately 20 minutes
Objective: Power/Coordination

Warm-up:
1 minute of Running
1 minute of Skipping
1 minute of Side Stepping

TEN 90-SECOND STATIONS:
1. Crab Walking
2. Balance Ball Crunches
3. Burpies
4. V Ups
5. Zig Zags
6. Balance Ball Chest Lifts
7. Box Jumps
8. Insects
9. Body Lifts
10. Plank

Cool down:
2 minutes of Walking

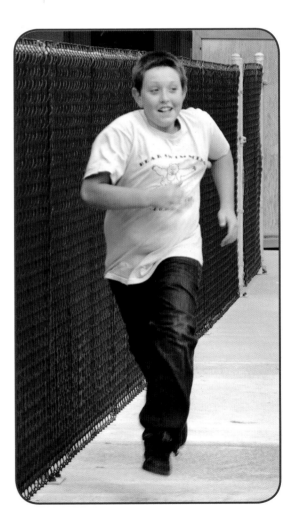

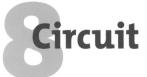

Circuit

Approximately 20 minutes
Objective: Power/Coordination

Warm-up:
3 minutes of Running

TEN 90-SECOND STATIONS:
1. Alternating Extensions
2. Bleacher Dips
3. Hula Hoop
4. V Ups
5. Plank
6. Balance Ball Chest Lifts
7. One Leg Balancing
   (left then right)
8. Leg Lifts
9. Medicine Ball Squats
10. Balance Ball Passes

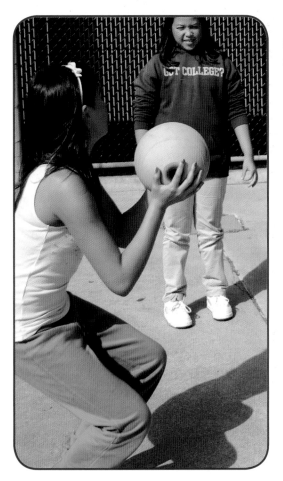

Cool down:
2 minutes of Walking

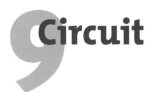

9 Circuit

Approximately 20 minutes
Objective: Power/Stability

Warm-up:
1 minute of Jump Rope
1 minute of Arm Circles (left then right)
1 minute of Cherry Pickers

TEN 90-SECOND STATIONS:
1. Streamlined Leaps
2. Body Lifts
3. Left, Right, Ups
4. Speed Jump Rope
5. Corner Push Outs
6. Plank
7. Squats
8. Hand Switch
9. Balance Ball Crunches
10. Air Kicking

Cool down:
2 minutes of Walking

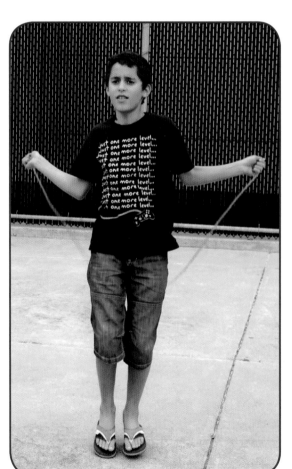

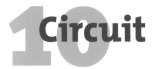Circuit

Approximately 20 minutes
Objective: Power/Tempo

Warm-up:
3 minutes of Stairs

TEN 90-SECOND STATIONS:
1. Speed Jump Roping
2. Bleacher Dips
3. Box Jumps
4. Plank
5. Balance Ball Chest Lifts
6. Air Kicking
7. Bleacher Dips
8. Balance Ball Crunches
9. Lunges
10. Hula Hoop

Cool down:
2 minutes of Walking

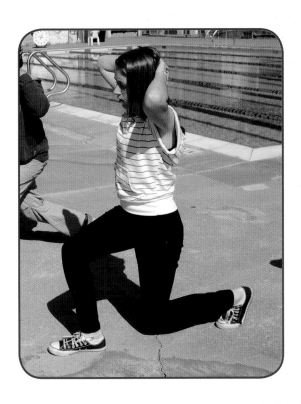

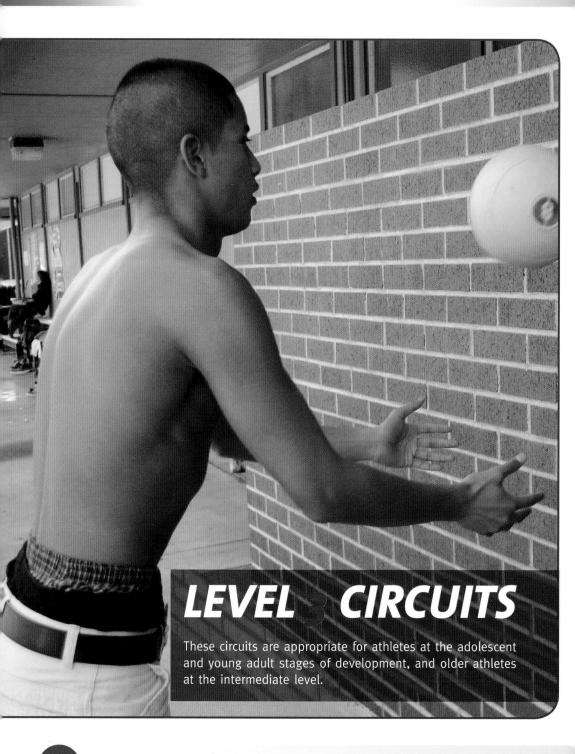

LEVEL 3 CIRCUITS

These circuits are appropriate for athletes at the adolescent and young adult stages of development, and older athletes at the intermediate level.

11 Circuit

Approximately 30 minutes
Objective: Power/Tempo

Warm-up:
1 minute of Arm Circles (left then right)
3 minutes of Stairs
3 minutes of Running Lines

TEN 2-MINUTE STATIONS:
1. Double Arm Pull with Stretch Cord
2. Standing Wall Rebounds with Medicine Ball
3. Box Jumps
4. Figure Eights with Medicine Ball
5. Double Arm Triceps Press with Stretch Cord
6. Twists with Medicine Ball
7. Alternating Arm Pull with Stretch Cord
8. Squats with Medicine Ball
9. Plank and Side Plank (left and right)
10. V Ups

Cool down:
3 minutes of Walking

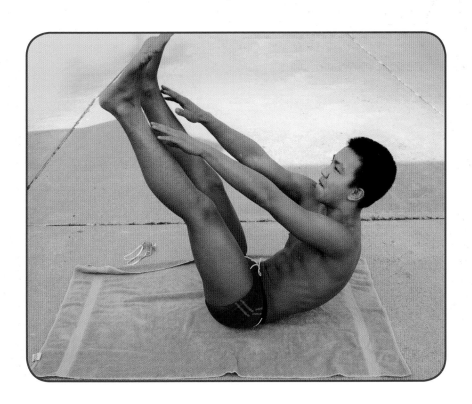

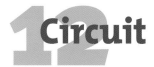Circuit

Approximately 30 minutes
Objective: Power/Stability

Warm-up:
3 minutes of Running
2 minutes of Burpies
2 minutes of Skipping

TEN 90-SECOND STATIONS
1. Peg Board
2. Double Arm Pull with Stretch Cord
3. Box Jumps
4. Squats with Medicine Ball
5. Plank, Side Plank - left then right
6. Left, Right, Ups with Medicine Ball
7. Alternating Arm Pull with Stretch Cord
8. Bar Dips
9. rog Jumps
10. Lunges with Medicine Ball

Cool down:
3 minutes of Walking

13 Circuit

Approximately 30 minutes
Objective: Power/Coordination/Explosiveness

Warm-up:
3 minutes of Stairs
1 minute of Burpies
3 minutes of Jump Rope

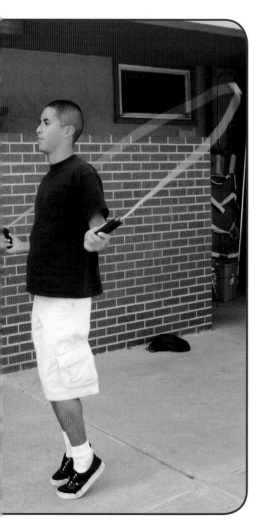

TEN 90-SECOND STATIONS:
1. Rope Climbing
2. Standing Wall Rebounds with Medicine Ball
3. Plank
4. Double Arm Pull with Stretch Cord
5. Leg Lift and Pass
6. Alternating Arm Pull with Stretch Cord
7. Squat and Jump with Medicine Ball
8. Balance Ball Passes
9. Double Arm Triceps Press with Stretch Cord
10. Speed Jump Rope

Cool down:
3 minutes of Walking

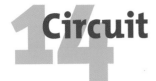

Circuit

Approximately 30 minutes
Objective: Power

Warm-up:
1 minute of Quick Clap
2 minutes of Jumping Jacks
3 minutes of Stairs
1 minute of Zig Zags

TEN 90-SECOND STATIONS:
1. Insect
2. Balance Ball Crunches
3. Bar Dips
4. Body Lifts
5. Squats with Medicine Ball
6. Speed Jump Rope
7. Double Arm Pull with Stretch Cord
8. Figure Eights with Medicine Ball
9. Plank, side Plank (left and right)
10. Medicine Ball Crunches

Cool down:
3 minutes of Walking

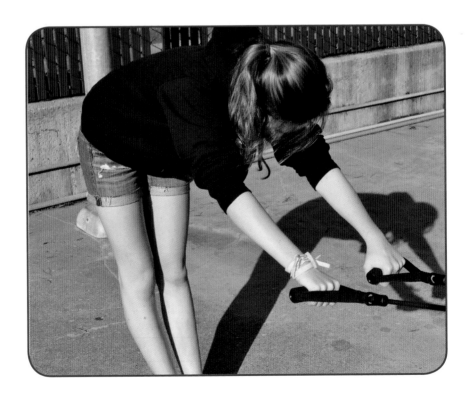

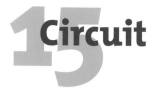

Circuit

Approximately 30 minutes
Objective: Power/Stability

Warm-up:
5 minutes of Running
1 minute of Hand Switches
1 minute of Cherry Pickers

TEN 90-SECOND STATIONS:
1. Corner Push Outs
2. Sky Crunches
3. Lunges with Medicine Ball
4. Body Lifts
5. Alternating Extensions
6. Bleacher Dips
7. Balance Ball Chest Lifts
8. Double Arm Pull with Stretch Cord
9. Leg Crosses
10. Peg Board

Cool down:
3 minutes of Walking

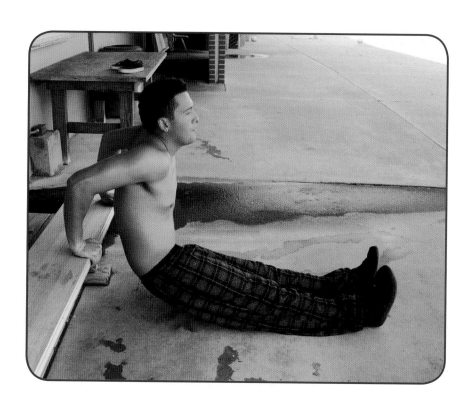

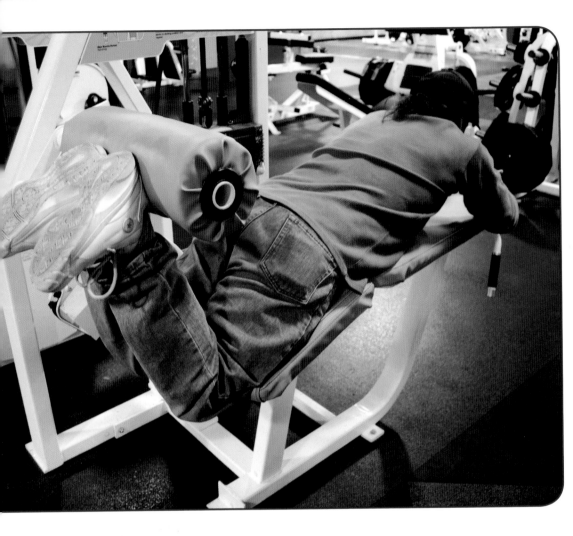

LEVEL 4 CIRCUITS

These circuits are appropriate for athletes at the young adult and adult stage of development.

16 Circuit

Approximately 1 hour
Objective: Power/Force

Warm-up:
15 minutes on Exercise Bike

Cool down:
5 minutes of Walking

TEN 2-MINUTE STATIONS.
(GO AROUND TWICE):
1. Lat Pull
2. Leg Press
3. March
4. Cable Pull
5. Hamstring Press
6. Incline Crunches
7. Triceps Extension
8. Bar Squats
9. Plank
10. Dumbbell Step Ups

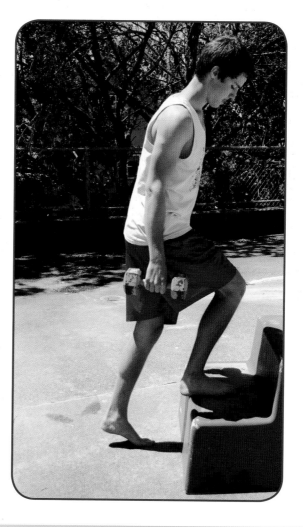

17 Circuit

Approximately 1 hour
Objective: Power/Force

Warm-up:
15 minutes on Elliptical Trainer

Cool down:
5 minutes of Walking

**TEN 2-MINUTE STATIONS
(GO AROUND TWICE):**

1. Bar Twists
2. Lat Pull
3. Incline Crunches
4. Standing Wall Rebounds with Medicine Ball
5. Triceps Extensions
6. Hamstring Lift
7. Double Arm Pull with Stretch Cord
8. Frog Jumps
9. Plank, Side Plank (left then right)
10. Rope Climbing

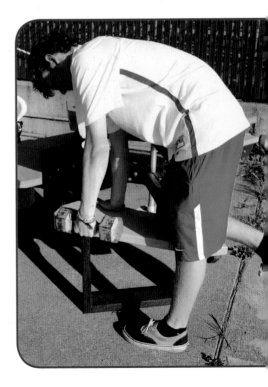

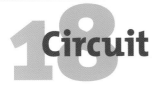

18 Circuit

Approximately 1 hour
Objective: Power/Force

Warm-up:
15 minutes on Elliptical Trainer

TEN 2-MINUTE STATIONS. (GO AROUND TWICE):
1. Bar Twists
2. March
3. Incline Crunches
4. Erg
5. Toe Raises with Bar
6. Curls
7. Alternating Extensions
8. Frog Jumps
9. Lunges with Dumbbells
10. Bar Dips

Cool down:
5 minutes of Walking

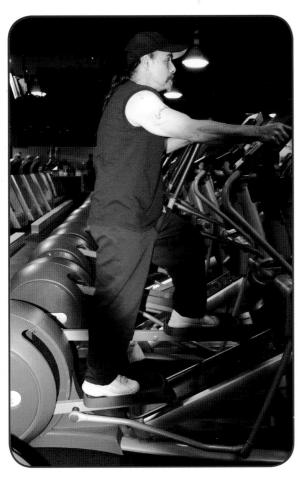

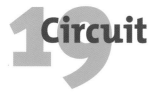
Circuit 19

Approximately 1 hour
Objective: Force/Explosiveness

Warm-up:
15 minutes on Exercise Bike

TEN 2-MINUTE STATIONS.
(GO AROUND TWICE):
1. Figure Eights with Medicine Ball
2. Double Arm Pull with Stretch Band
3. Lunges with Medicine Ball
4. Left Right, Ups with Medicine Ball
5. Leg Press
6. Lat Pull
7. V Ups
8. Frog Jumps
9. Erg
10. March

Cool down:
5 minutes of Walking

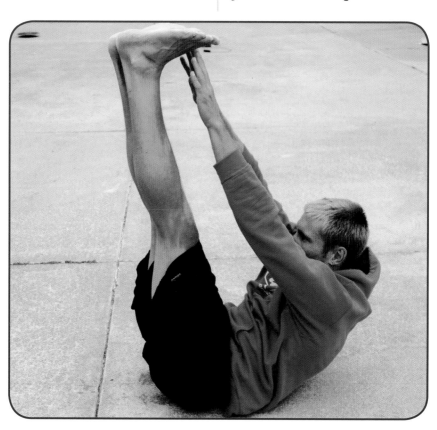

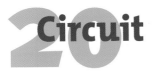

Circuit 20

Approximately 1 hour
Objective: Power/Stability

Warm-up:
15 minutes of Running

TEN 2-MINUTE STATIONS.
(GO AROUND TWICE):
1. March
2. Cable Pull
3. Alternating Extensions
4. Frog Jumps
5. Lat Pull
6. Triceps Press
7. Incline Crunches
8. Leg Press
9. Stretch Cord – Double Arm Pull
10. Balance Ball Chest Lifts

Cool down:
5 minutes of Walking

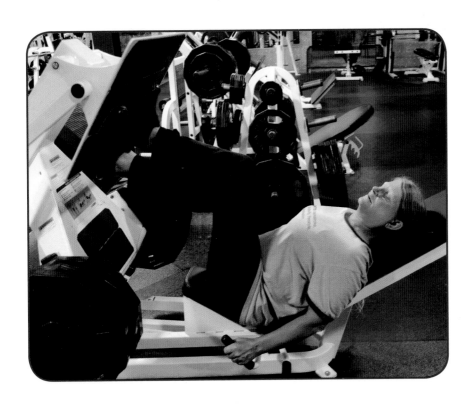

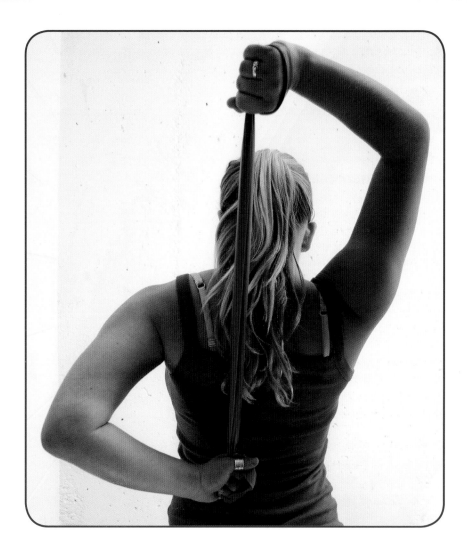

Shoulder Maintenance Routine

This exercise routine is designed to maintain and build shoulder stability for swimmers. It can be done every other day in addition to other strength training activities. Along with a stretch band, a small weight is required. Make sure each exercise is done with correct form as described on pages 65, 82-83, and 94-95. These exercises, done on an ongoing basis, will encourage balanced shoulder stability and strength in the most crucial and vulnerable swimming joints. If one or more of these exercises causes immediate pain, skip it and go on to the others. Give the skipped exercise another try each time this routine is done.

Shoulder Maintenance Routine

Warm-up:
1 minute of Hanging Circles (left arm)
1 minute of Hanging Circles (right arm)

12 x External Sweep (right arm)
12 x External Sweep (left arm)
12 x Internal Sweep (right arm)
12 x Internal Sweep (left arm)

1 minute of Corner Press
12 x Diagonal Lift (left arm)
12 x Diagonal Lift (right arm)

12 x Raise a Glass (left arm)
12 x Raise a Glass (right arm)
12 x Back Scrubbing (left arm high)
12 x Back Scrubbing (right arm high)

Cool down:
2 minutes of Walking

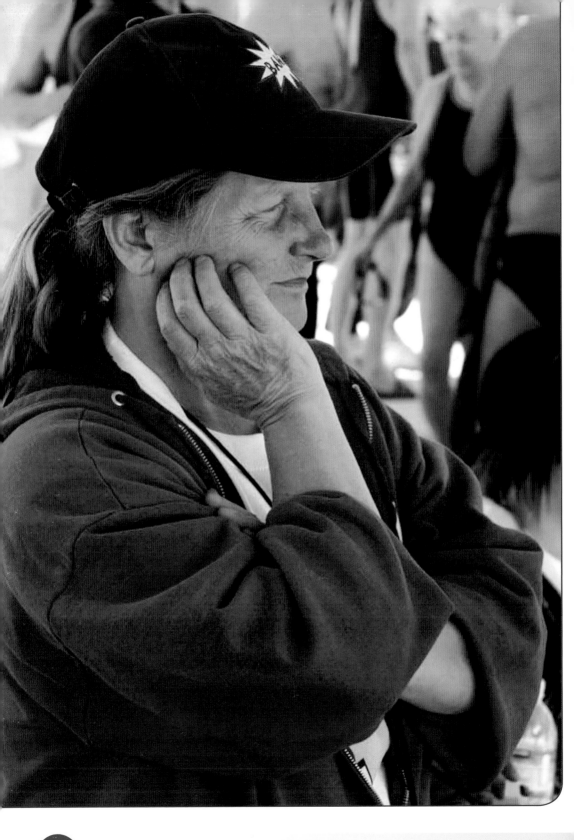

8 MEASURING PROGRESS

How do we know if our strength training is working? Ultimately, over time, we should see results in the pool. But we should also see progress within our strength work. Recording various exercises that are done regularly in terms of load, number of repetitions and sets and rate will allow us to track our progress.

The Strength Training Log presented on page 162 provides a basic structure for tracking progress. Make copies and use one sheet per month to record your strength training progress over time. At the beginning of each month, fill in the exercises that you will track on the left side of the page. Then, after each strength training session throughout the month, record your results for those exercises. Record the number of sets, repetitions or other information specific to the exercise for comparison.

At the end of the month, do a test set to gauge adaptation. A test set takes three of the exercises you have been doing throughout the month and increases the difficulty of each. The exact way the difficulty is increased depends on the objective. For instance, if your objective is more force, more load would be attempted. If your objective is tempo, more repetitions would be attempted in a fixed time. At the bottom of the Progress Log, a space is provided to record the results of a monthly test set.

If test set results show that you are able to perform the exercises with increased difficulty, then as you begin a new month of strength training, use the test set degree of difficulty as your new base.

Remember to focus on your objective. If you are training for more force, don't expect to see much progress in terms of number of repetitions. Look instead for progress in terms of amount of resistance. If you are training for more power, don't expect to see much progress in terms of the load. Look instead for rate, or number of repetitions.

Progress tracked that does not meet the objective, should be watched closely over several more weeks. Random progress across the board can be expected, but a trend of progress toward other than the strength objective indicates some change in the training content or routine is needed.

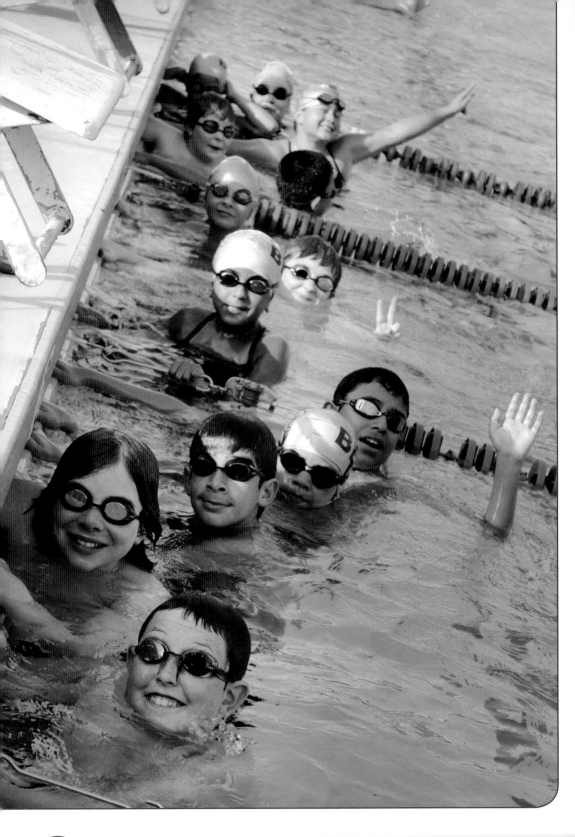

CONCLUSION

As you embark on a strength training program with the goal of achieving more swimming speed, please keep this thought in your mind. To become a fast swimmer, you have to be prepared to sow before you reap. Swimming is a sport that takes a lot of dedication over time. Day after day, you have to believe that all your training will pay off. Month after month, you have to have faith that you are developing in the right direction. Year after year, you have to trust that your ultimate swimming goal will be realized.

In this age of immediate gratification, swimmers have to be so patient! So, as you catch the next medicine ball, or make your way around the next circuit, take pride in your dedication and enjoy the process of moving toward your goal.

STRENGTH TRAINING PROGRESS LOG

Name _____

Month/Year _____

Exercise	Objective	Date / Results	Date / Results	Date / Results	Date / Results	Date / Results	Date / Results	Date / Results	Date / Results	Date / Results	Date / Results	Date / Results	Date / Results
SELF RESISTANCE													
1.													
2.													
3.													
4.													
5.													
MEDICINE BALL													
1.													
2.													
3.													
4.													
STRETCH CORD													
1.													
2.													
3.													
4.													
WEIGHTS													
1.													
2.													
3.													
4.													

MONTHLY TEST SET

Exercise	Objective	New Challenge	Results
1.			
2.			
3.			

CREDITS

Illustrations: Blythe Lucero

Photography: Blythe Lucero, Avital Brodin, Photo of seal courtesy of Andreas Trepte, www.photo-natur.de

Cover Photo: © Jupiterimages/2006 Comstock Images/Thinkstock
Jacket Photo: © iStockphoto/Thinkstock

Cover Design: Sabine Groten

Special thanks to the talented athletes of BEAR Swimming who are pictured in this book. They include: Josh Aiala, Nick Boss, Elliot Carr, Daniel Chavez, Darren Chavez, Alex Cortez, Biranya Cortez, Christian Cortez, William Cross, Esther Cuan, Jessica Eciso, Julio Eciso, Brayn Gomez, Natalie Gomez, Giovanni Hernandez, Jacob Malaga, Nicholas Malaga, Ziad Mosalam, Adrian Murillo and Diego Paucar.

Special thanks to the talented athletes of Berkeley Barracudas who are pictured in this book. They include: Isabel Augustine, Jennifer Barra, Katie Howard, Lydia Howard, Angelica Joseph, Juliana Price, Elliot Ngyun, Lydia Price, Zack Price, Victor Rivas, Morgan Rose, Sarah Tuma, Spencer Tuma and Robin Wampler.

Special thanks to the talented athletes of Berkeley Aquatic Masters who are pictured in this book. They include: Pam Bennett, Conny Bleul Gohlke, Jonas Brodin, Miriam Ciochon, Kathryn Cohen, Lessly Field, Seth Goddard, Tami Kasamatsu and Alvaro Pastor.

In addition, special thanks to the following individuals who are pictured in this book: Vince Corbella, Alyssa Perrucchi, Chris Fish, Siobhan Langlois, Bonnie Lucero, Eric Lucero, Grace Nelson-Barrer and Hans Tanalski.

INCREASE YOUR STRENGTH!

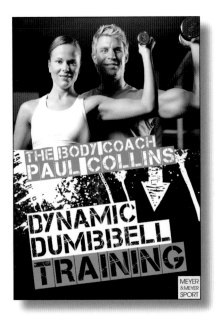

Paul Collins
Dynamic Dumbbell Training

Paul Collins' Dynamic Dumbbell Training and
3-Stage Dynamic Dumbbell Training System is
aimed at improving everyday lifestyle and athletic
movement patterns. Learn how to increase
muscular size, strength, balance and coordination
and explosive power for improving athletic
performance.

ISBN: 9781841263106
E-Book: 9781841267036
$ 18.95 US/$ 32.95 AUS
£ 14.95 UK/€ 18.95

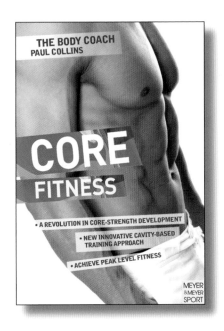

Paul Collins
Core Fitness

This training method allows you to fuse the trunk
muscles in co-contraction with the deeper
stabilizing muscles for better body awareness,
breathing efficiency, motor control and spinal
support in all movement patterns. A stronger core
translates to better overall athletic performance.

ISBN: 9781841262925
E-Book: 9781841265810
$ 14.95 US/$ 22.95 AUS
£ 9.95 UK/€ 14.95

All books available as ⊙**mediaTresor** E-books.
SECURE E-BOOK
- secure & user-friendly

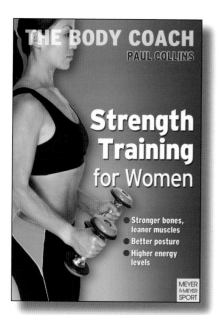

Paul Collins
Strength Training for Women

The combination of strength training, aerobic exercise and healthy eating habits has proven to be most effective for fat loss and muscle toning. This program has been developed as a training guide as more women begin to understand the health benefits of this activity.

ISBN: 9781841262482
E-Book: 9781841265483
$ 14.95 US/$ 22.95 AUS
£ 9.95 UK/€ 14.95

Paul Collins
Athletic Abs
Build Your Strongest Core Ever

Develop core strength, power and a rock-hard mid-section to help drive your athletic performance to a new level. This cutting edge training program combines a progressive series of abdominal strengthening exercises aimed at improving posture, body awareness, and motor control.

ISBN: 9781841262956
E-Book: 9781841265803
$ 14.95 US/$ 22.95 AUS
£ 9.95 UK/€ 14.95

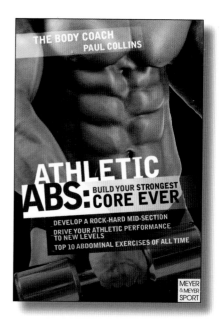

www.m-m-sports.com